Why Keisha wanted to become a Nurse

By

Valerie Clary Muronda

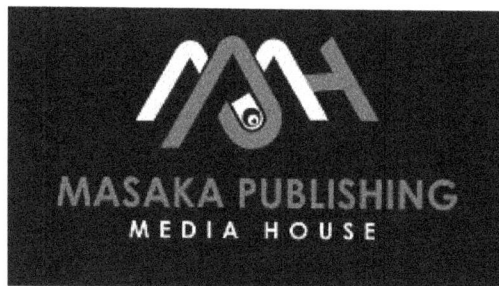

MASAKA PUBLISHING
MEDIA HOUSE

ISBN: 978-1-965398-37-1
©Valerie Clary Muronda
MASAKA PUBLISHING MEDIA HOUSE
alf@cp7sisters.com

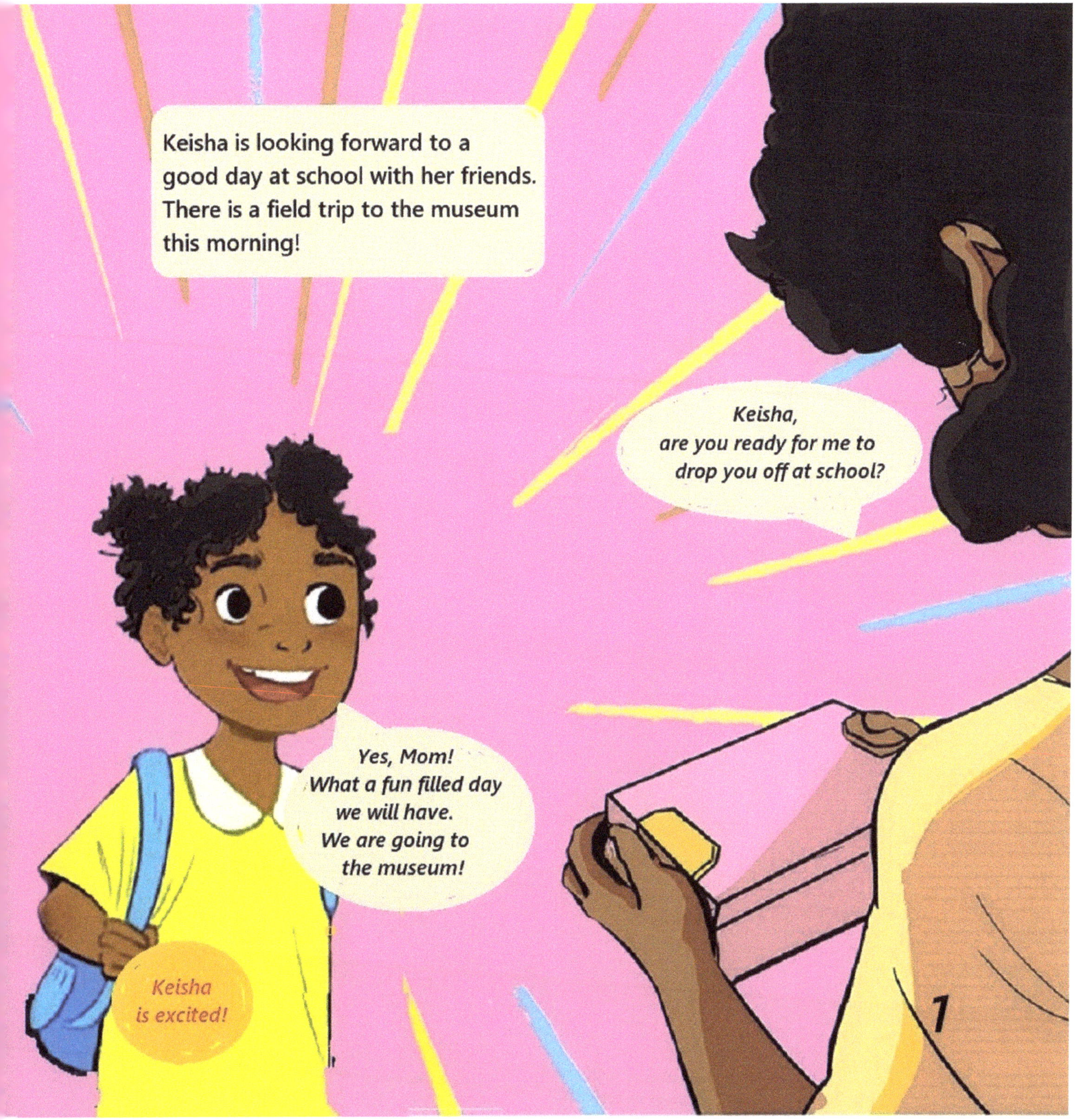
Keisha is looking forward to a good day at school with her friends. There is a field trip to the museum this morning!
Keisha, are you ready for me to drop you off at school?
Yes, Mom! What a fun filled day we will have. We are going to the museum!
Keisha is excited!

Keisha is excited to see her friends
Cathy, Carol and Dee.
They play and run around the school
yard until the first bell rings.

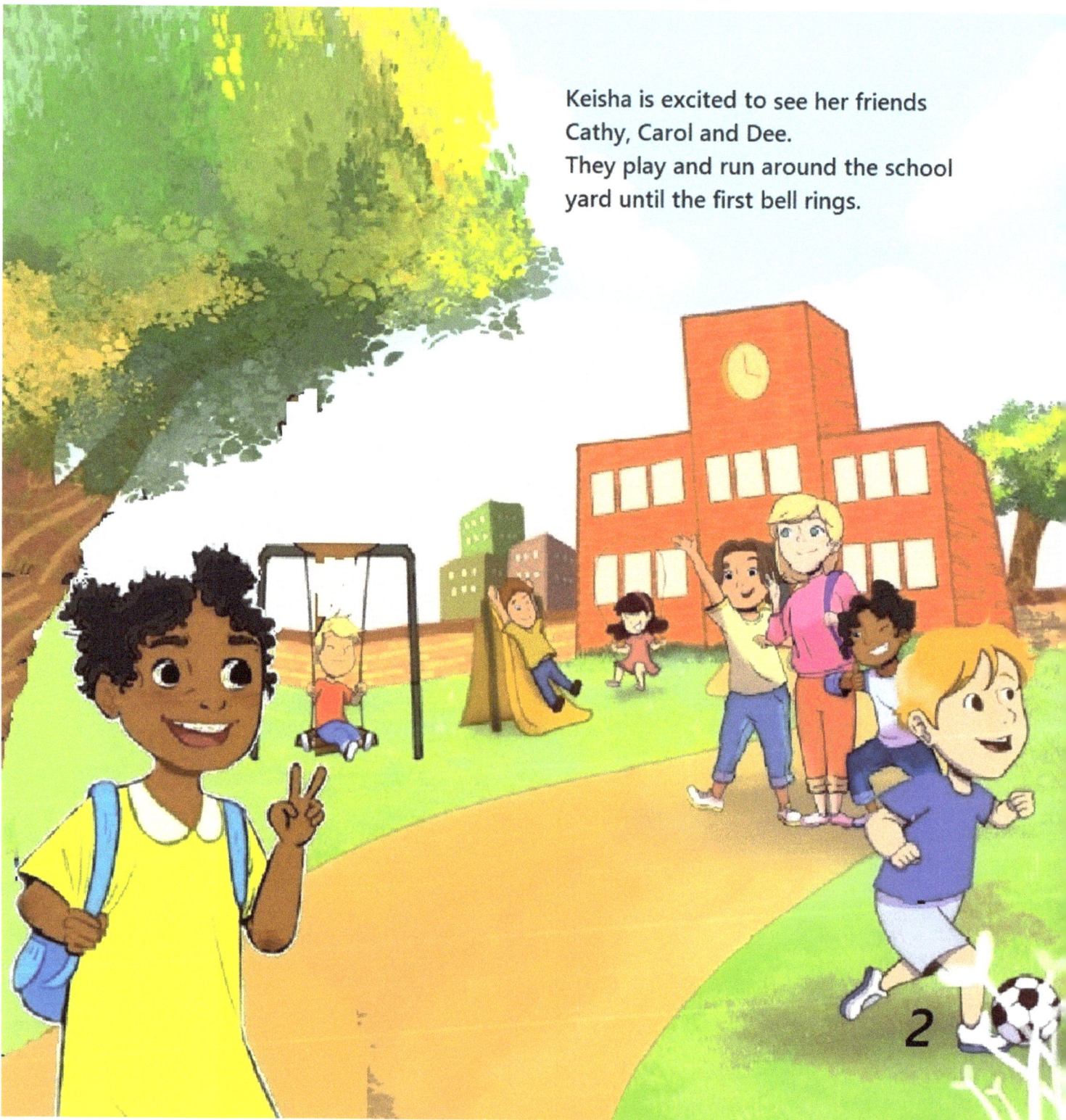

2

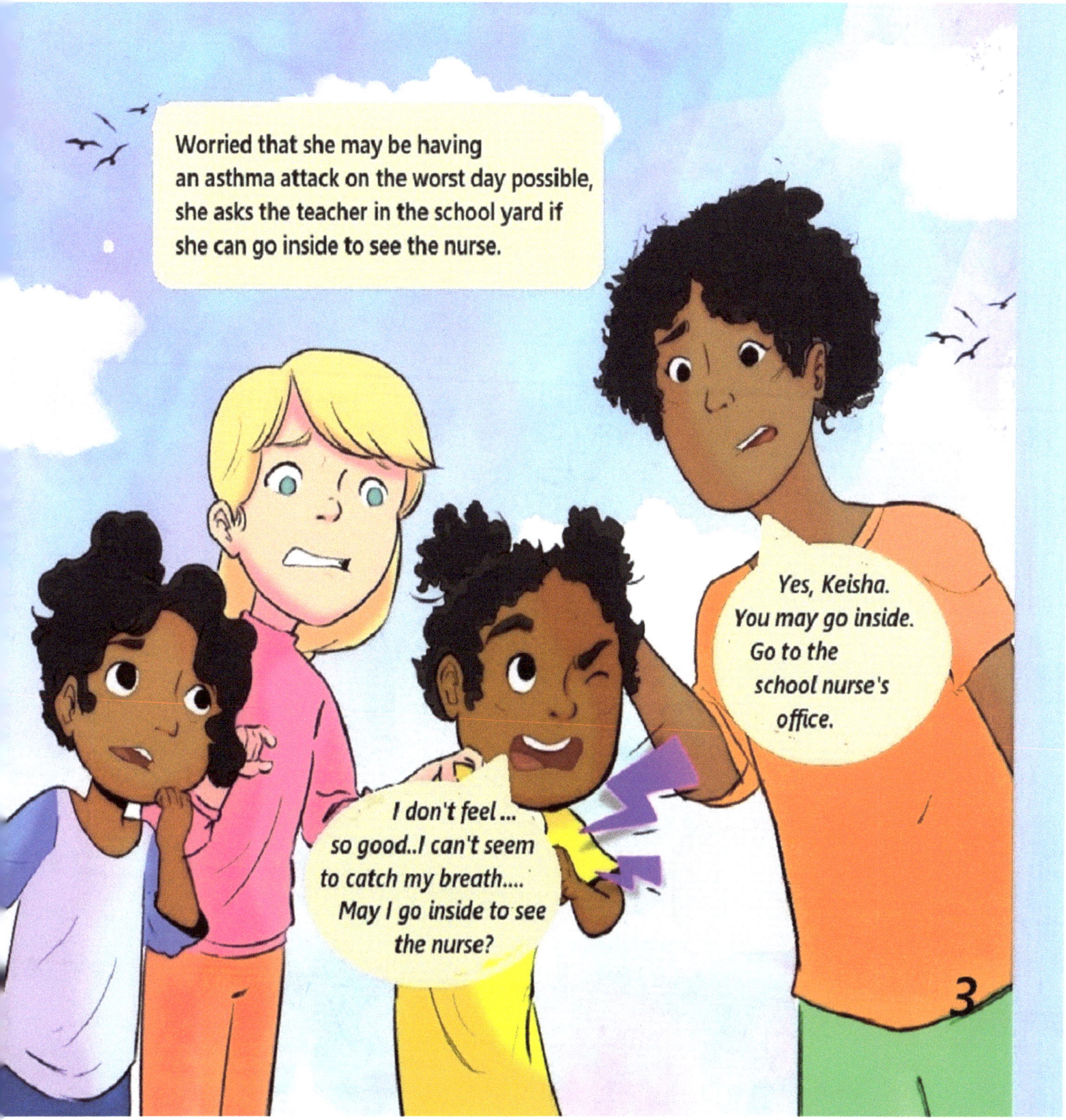
Worried that she may be having an asthma attack on the worst day possible, she asks the teacher in the school yard if she can go inside to see the nurse.
I don't feel ... so good..I can't seem to catch my breath.... May I go inside to see the nurse?
Yes, Keisha. You may go inside. Go to the school nurse's office.

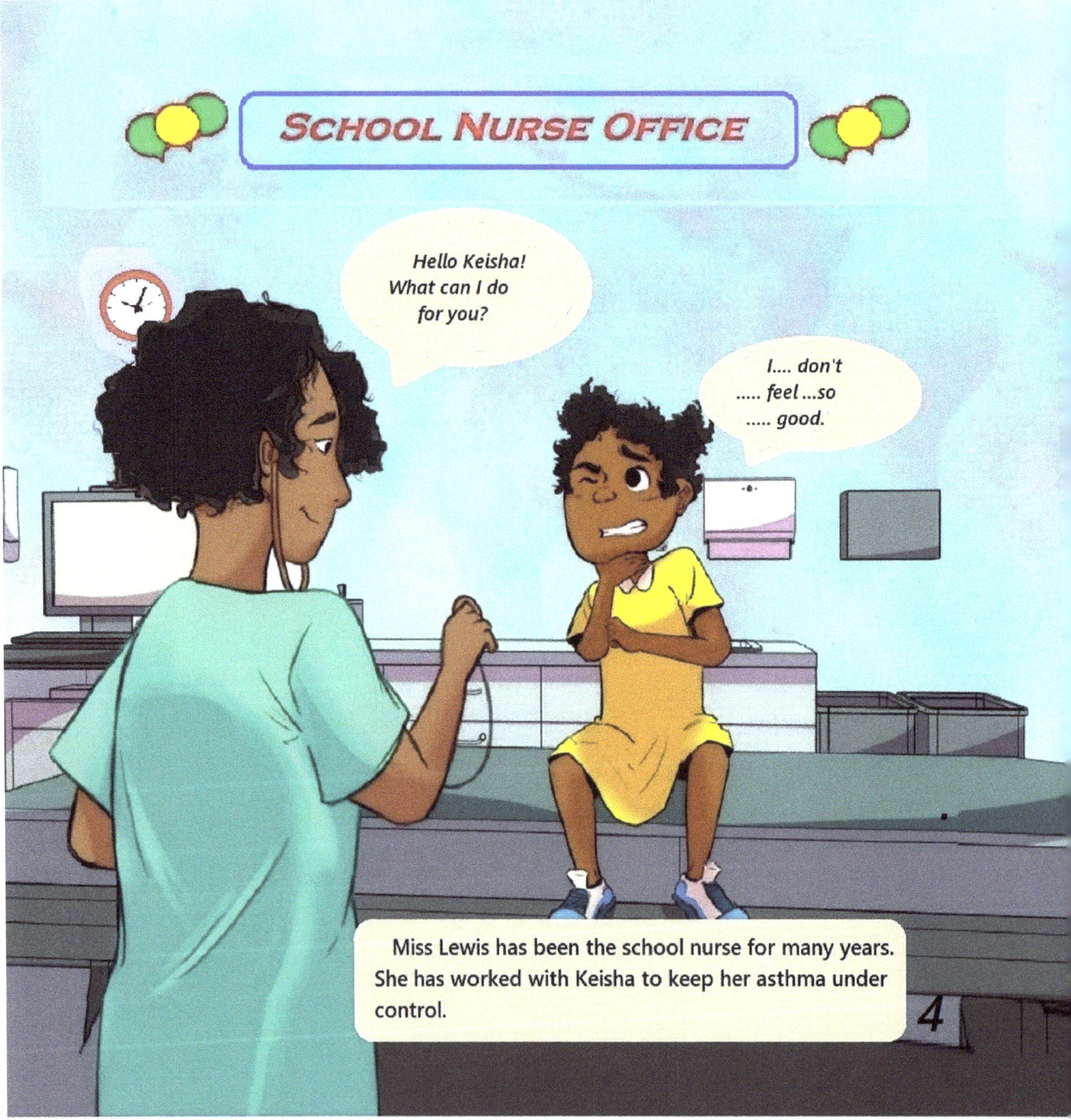
SCHOOL NURSE OFFICE
Hello Keisha! What can I do for you?
I.... don't ..... feel ...so ..... good.
Miss Lewis has been the school nurse for many years. She has worked with Keisha to keep her asthma under control.

SCHOOL NURSE OFFICE

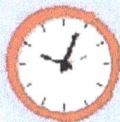

After she listens to Keisha's lungs with the s-t-e-t-h-o-s-c-o-p-e she looks at Keisha worriedly.

Okay, let's try a few things to see if we can get you breathing better.

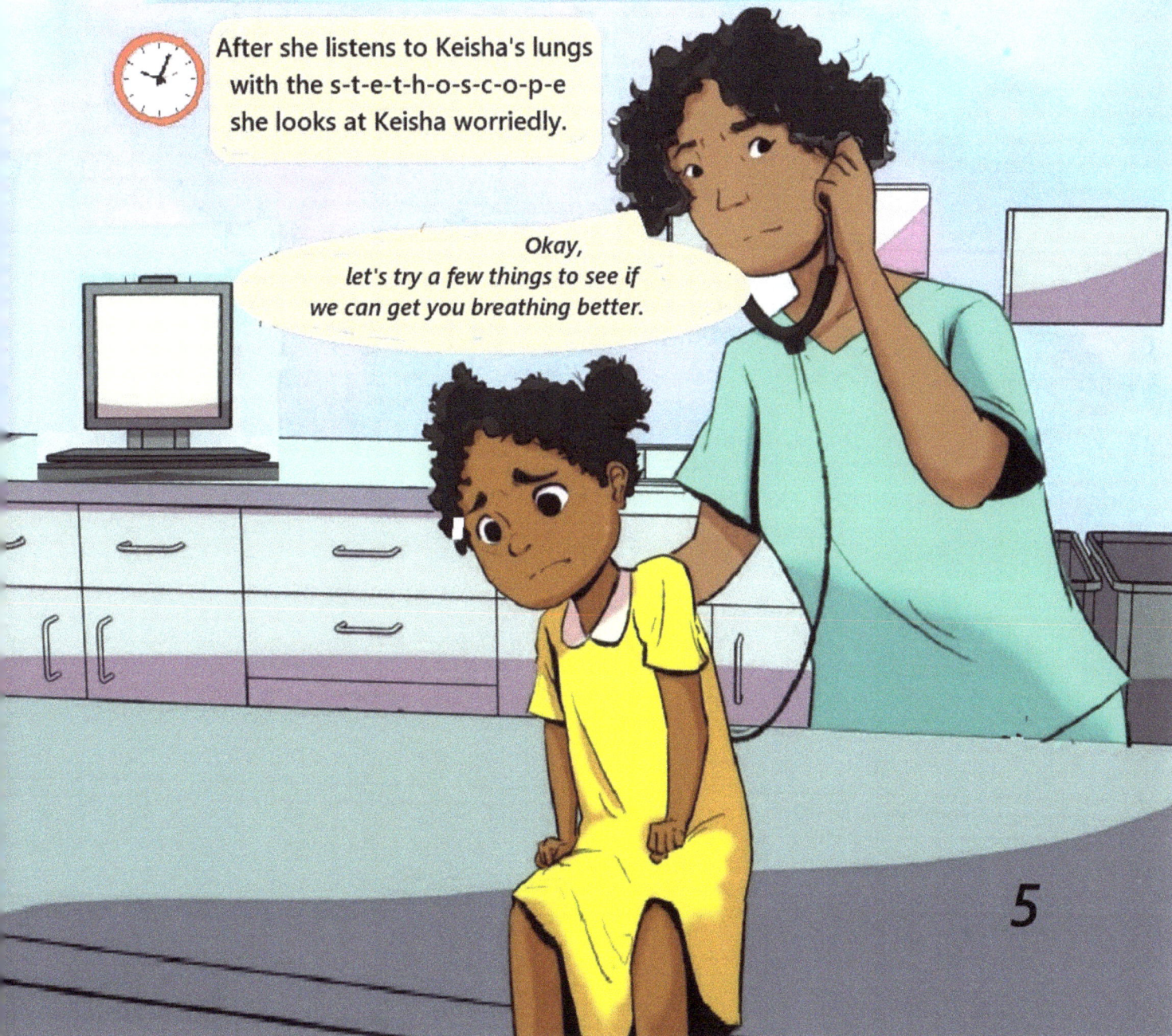

5

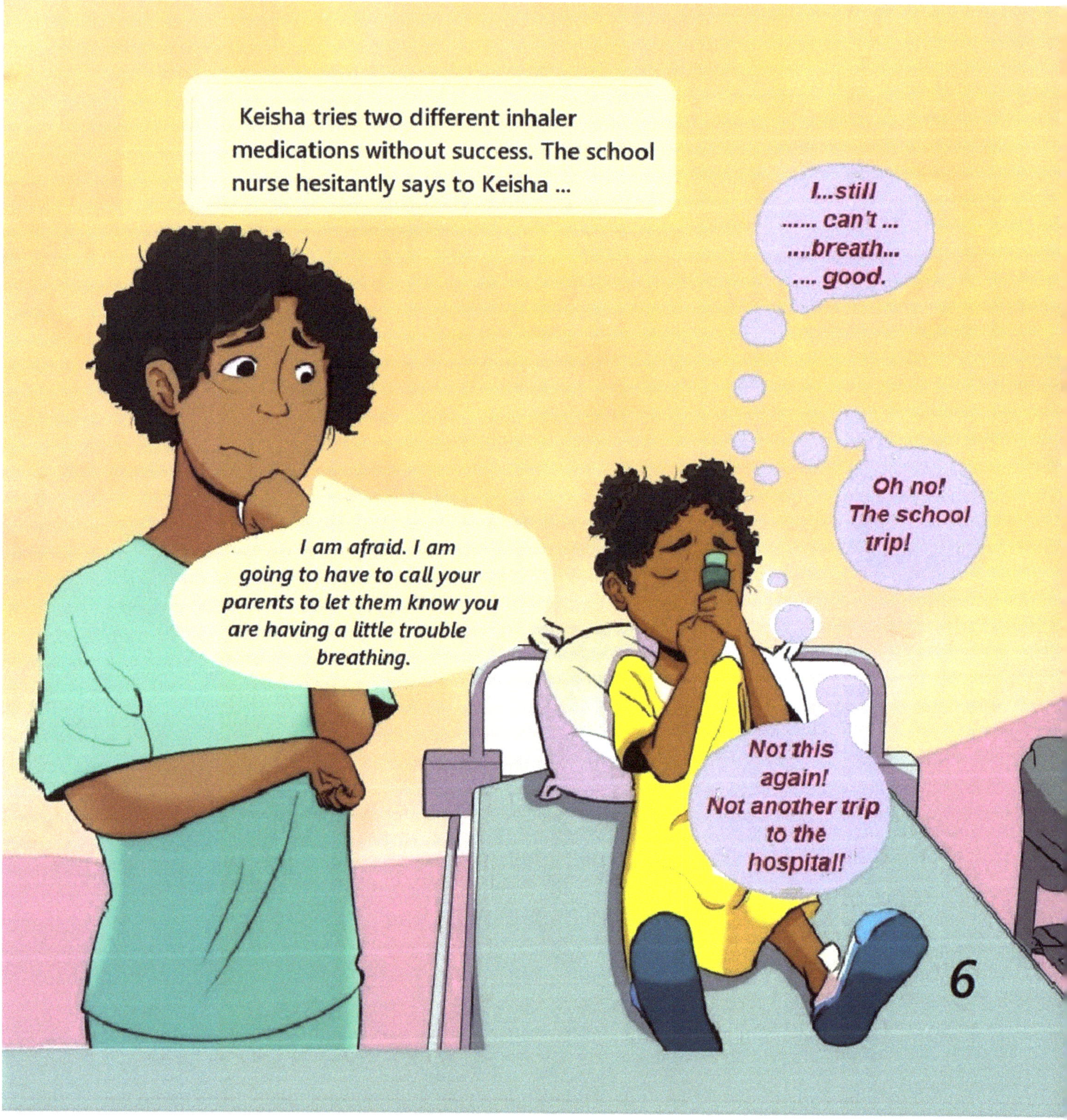
Keisha tries two different inhaler medications without success. The school nurse hesitantly says to Keisha ...
I am afraid. I am going to have to call your parents to let them know you are having a little trouble breathing.
I...still ...... can't ... .breath... .... good.
Oh no! The school trip!
Not this again! Not another trip to the hospital!

Keisha's dad
is here
to take her
to the hospital.

OXYGEN

The school nurse helps Keisha use two of her regular inhalers, and when that does not work, she gives Keisha a treatment.
By the worried look on the nurse's face, Keisha can tell, she is headed for another hospital stay. Again!

7

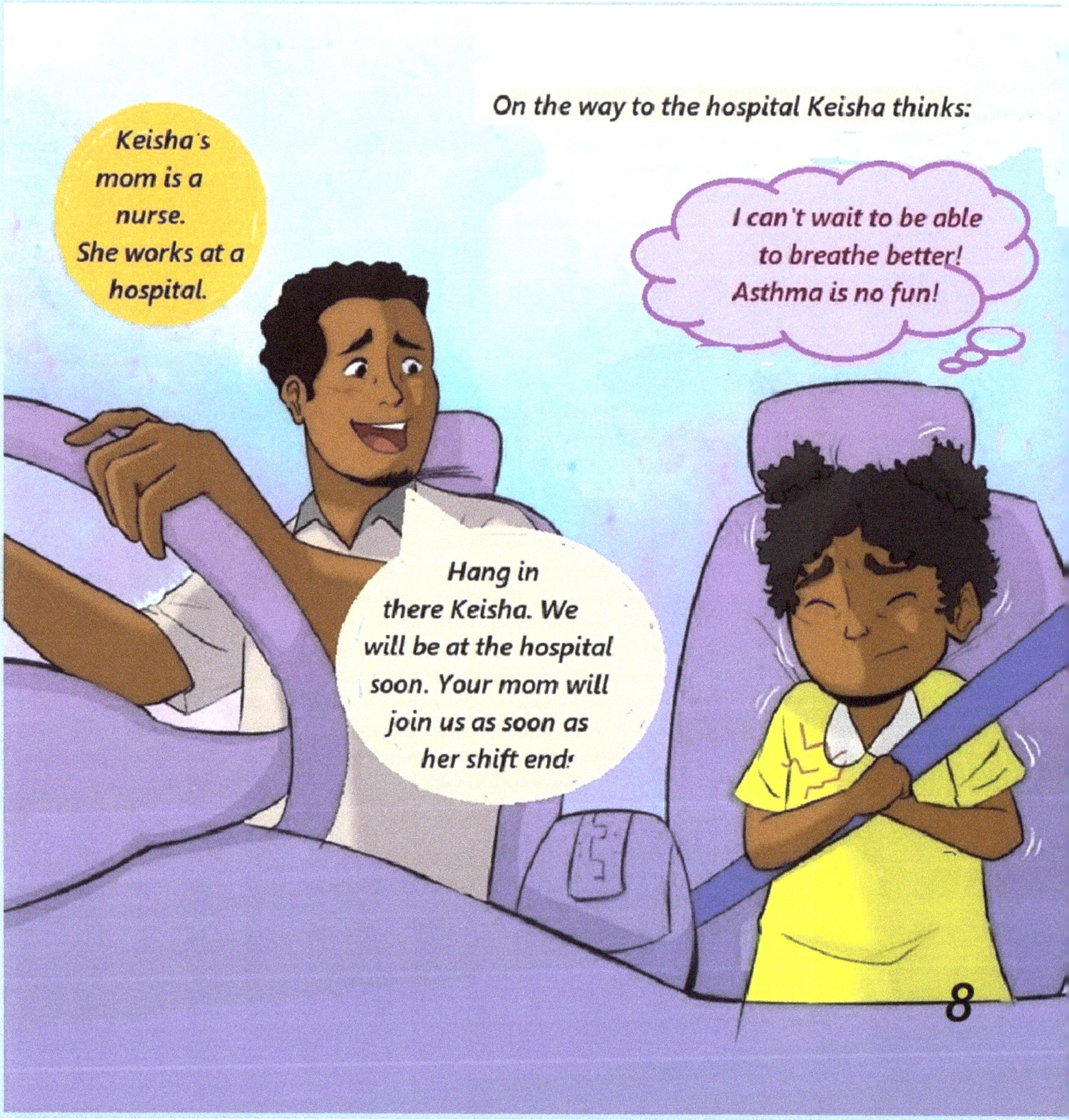
On the way to the hospital Keisha thinks:
Keisha's mom is a nurse. She works at a hospital.
I can't wait to be able to breathe better! Asthma is no fun!
Hang in there Keisha. We will be at the hospital soon. Your mom will join us as soon as her shift end

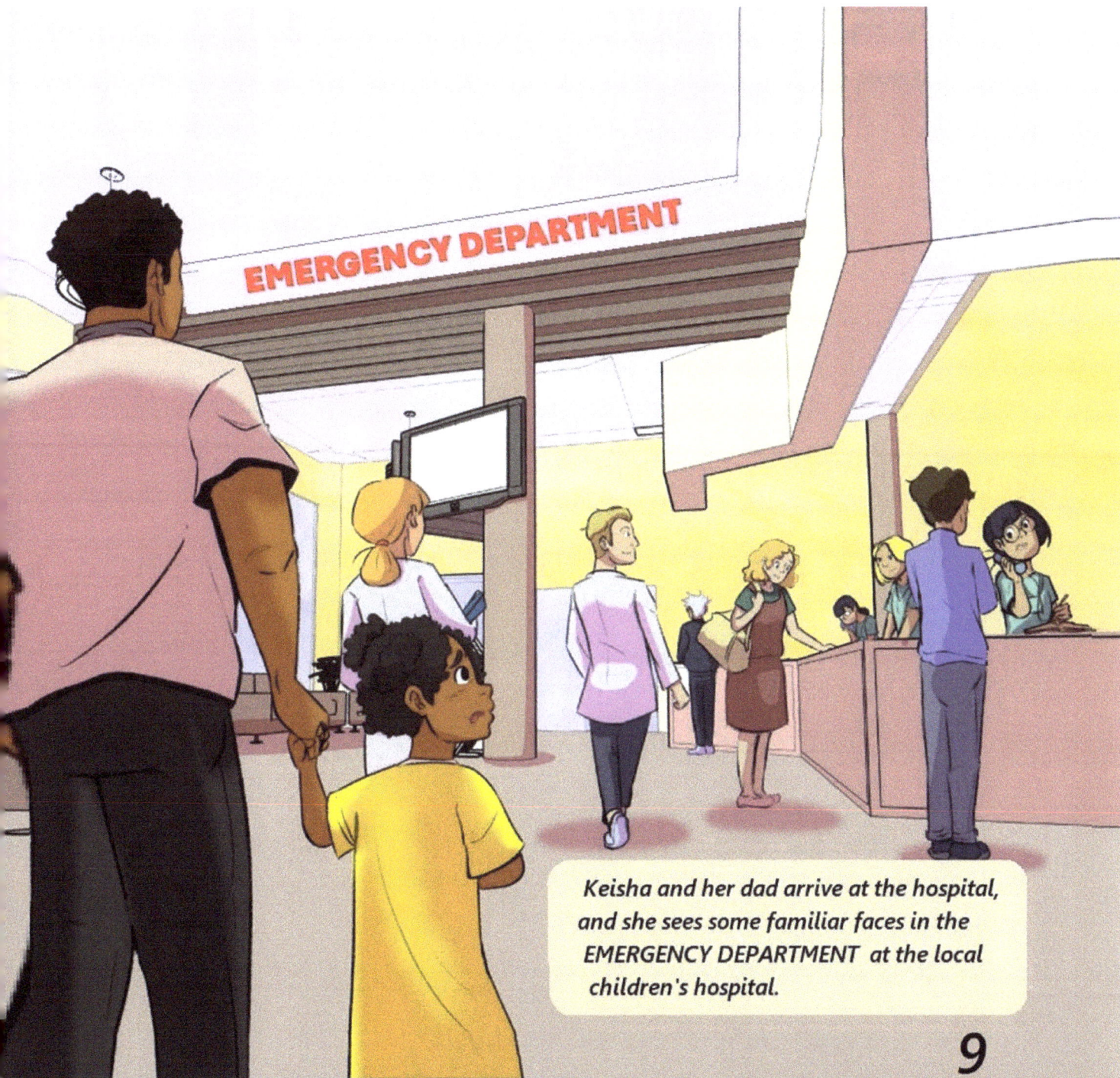

Keisha and her dad arrive at the hospital, and she sees some familiar faces in the EMERGENCY DEPARTMENT at the local children's hospital.

9

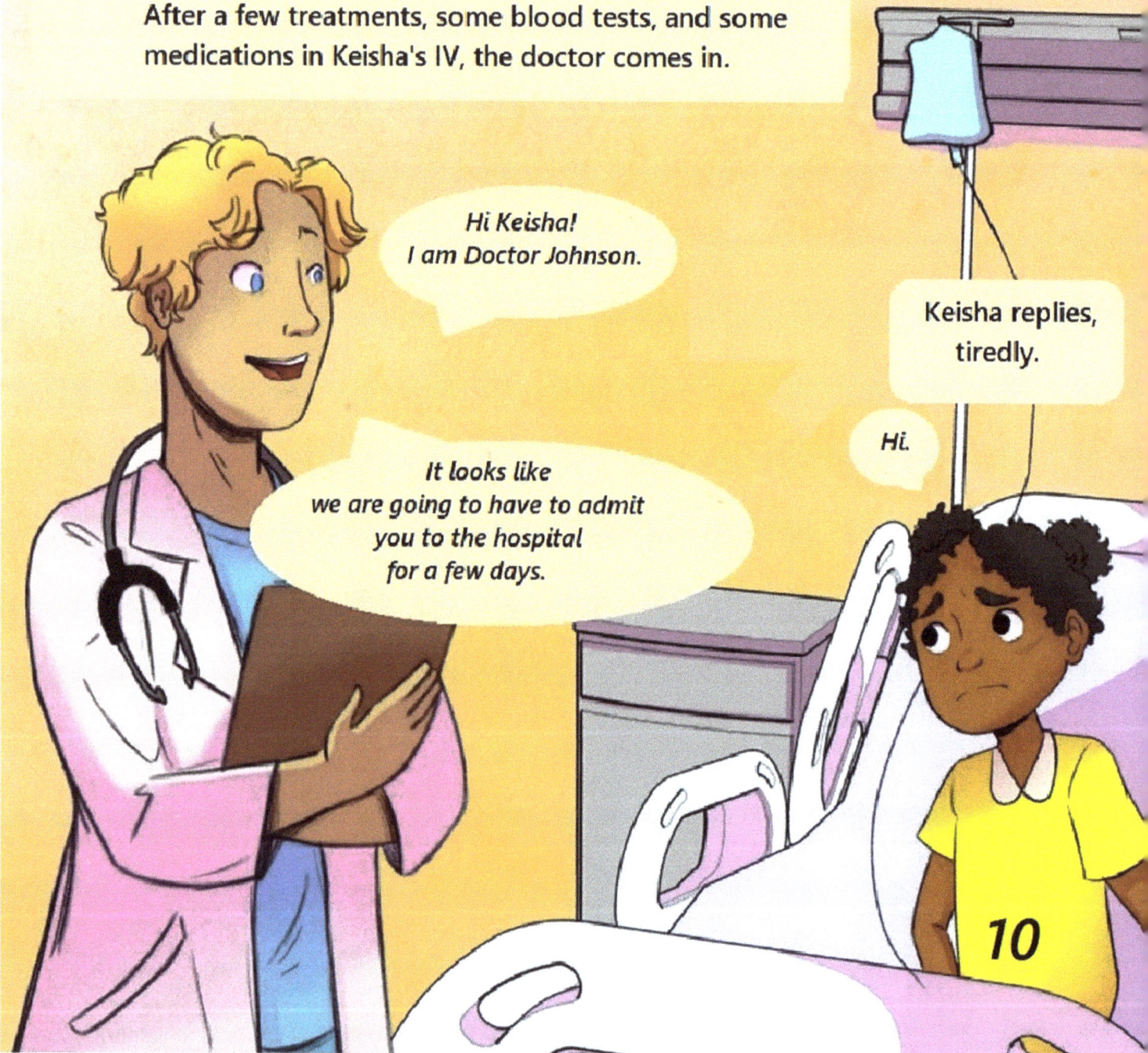

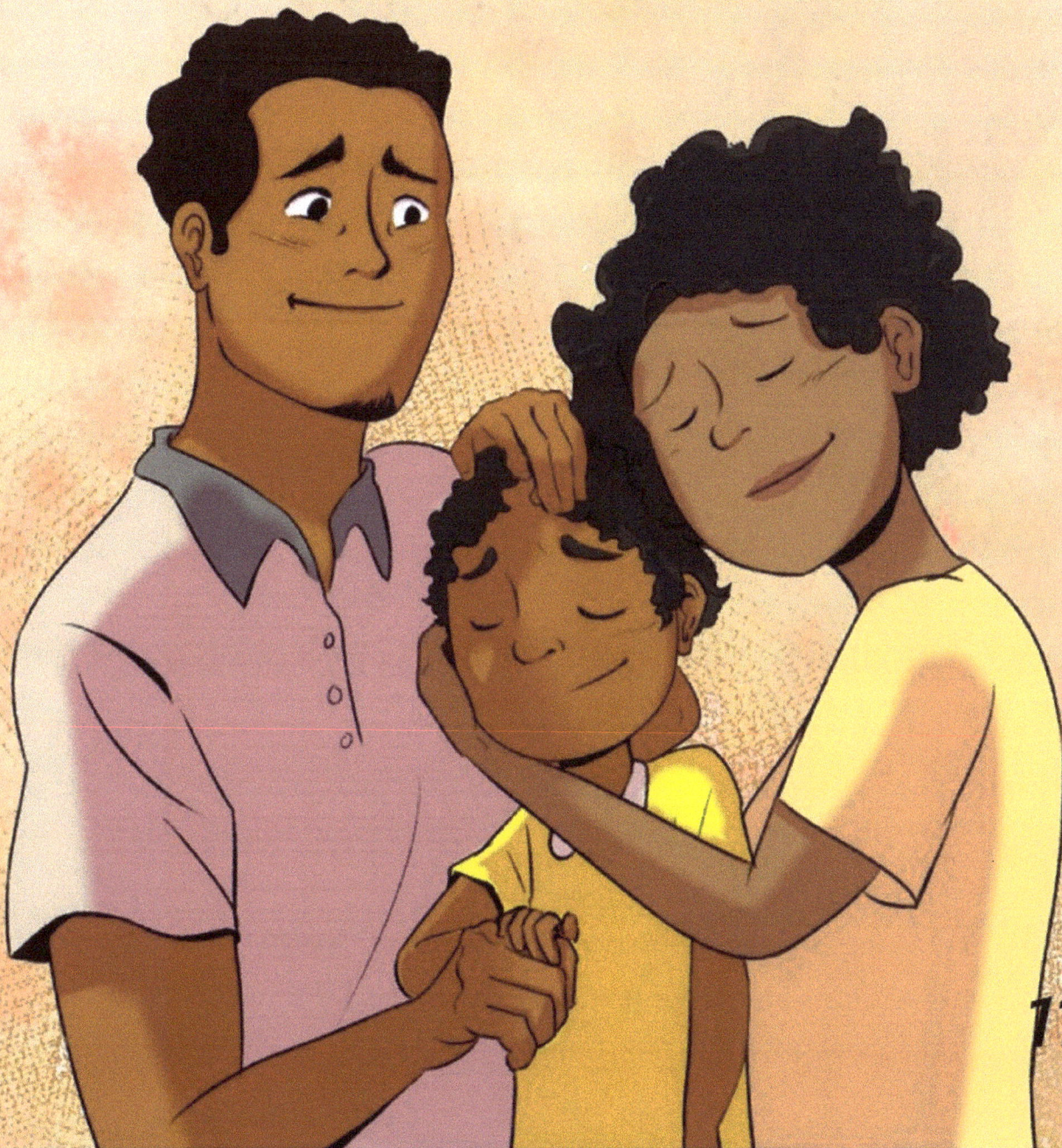

Both Keisha's parents, give Keisha a reassuring hug.

After a few hours in the Emergency
Department, Keisha is admitted to
her hospital room.

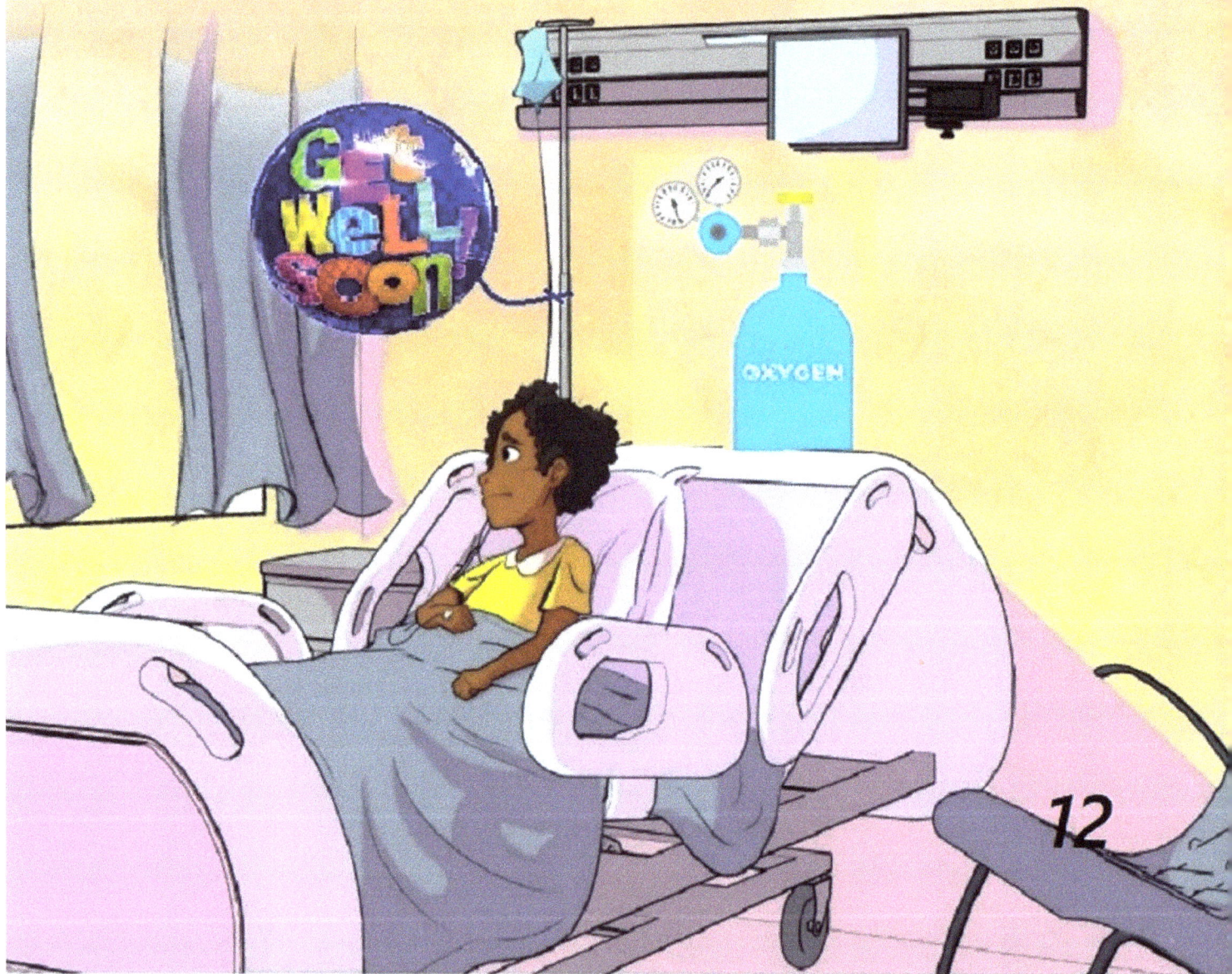

Keisha looks at the familiar unit she has been a patient on several times. Sleepily, Keisha wonders who her nurse will be. She knows many of the nurses here!

A few moments later, in walks Kadijah.

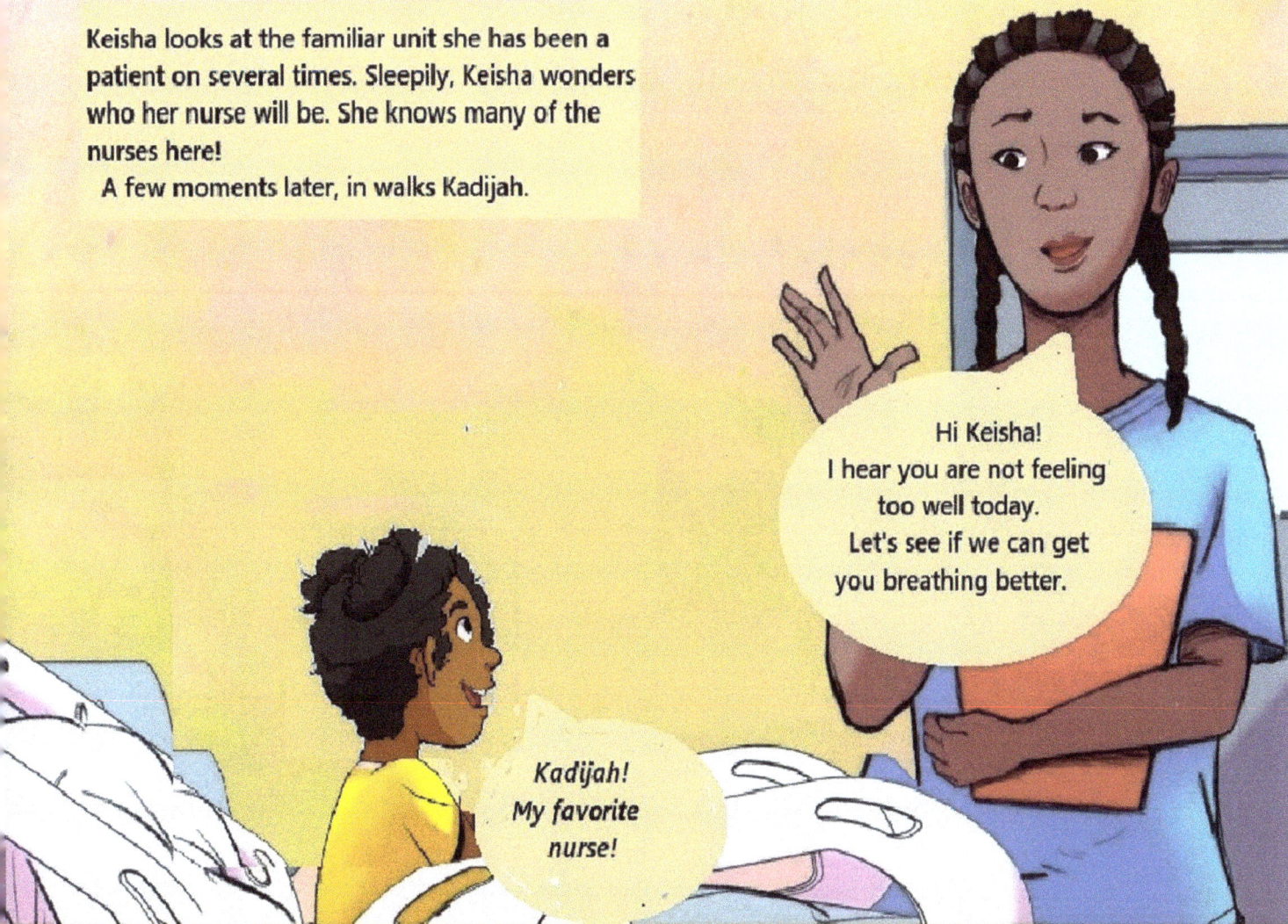

Hi Keisha! I hear you are not feeling too well today. Let's see if we can get you breathing better.

Kadijah! My favorite nurse!

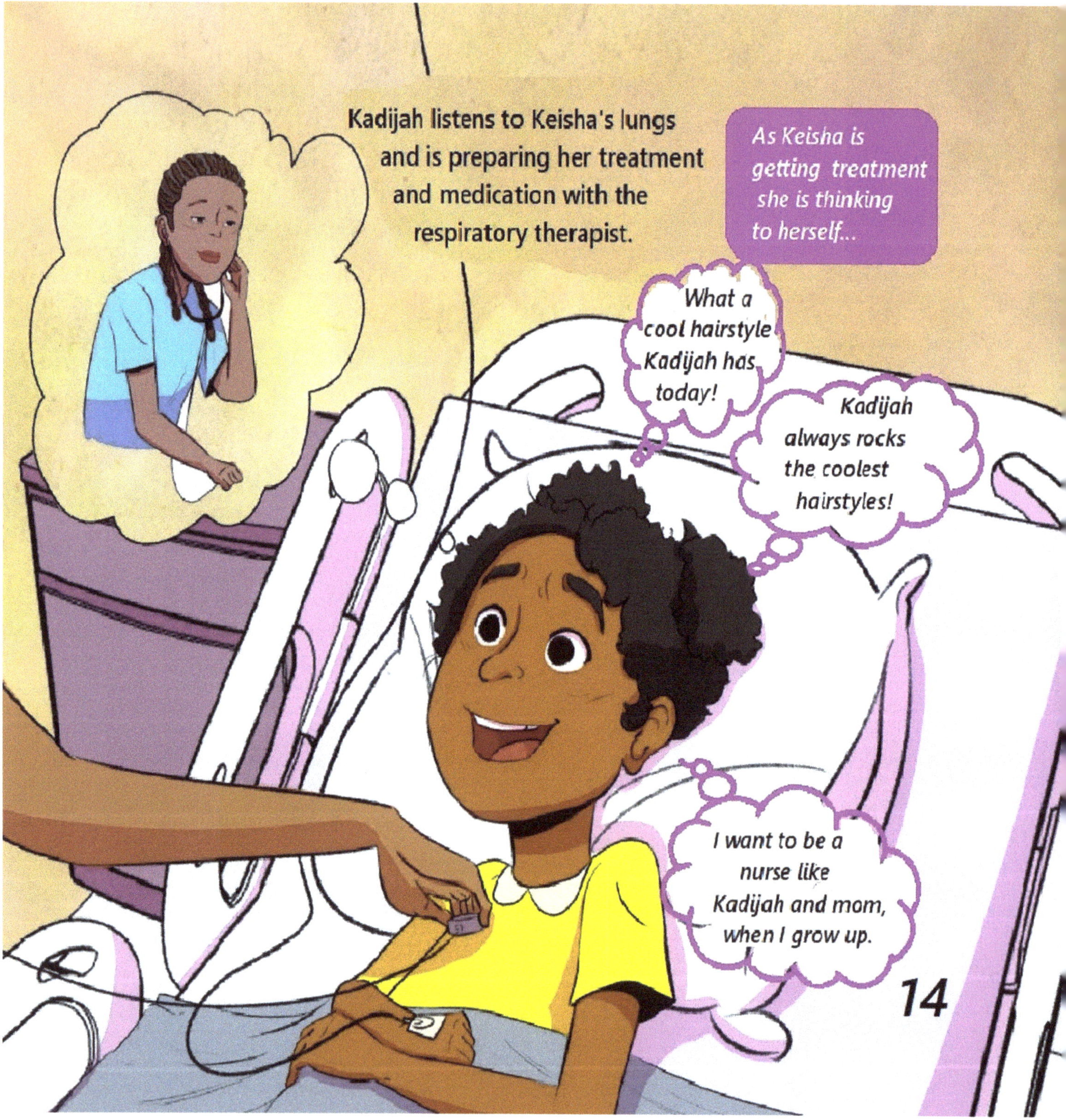
Kadijah listens to Keisha's lungs and is preparing her treatment and medication with the respiratory therapist.
As Keisha is getting treatment she is thinking to herself...
What a cool hairstyle Kadijah has today!
Kadijah always rocks the coolest hairstyles!
I want to be a nurse like Kadijah and mom, when I grow up.

After an afternoon of treatments and falling asleep napping, Keisha wakes up in the middle of the night.

She puts on the call light.

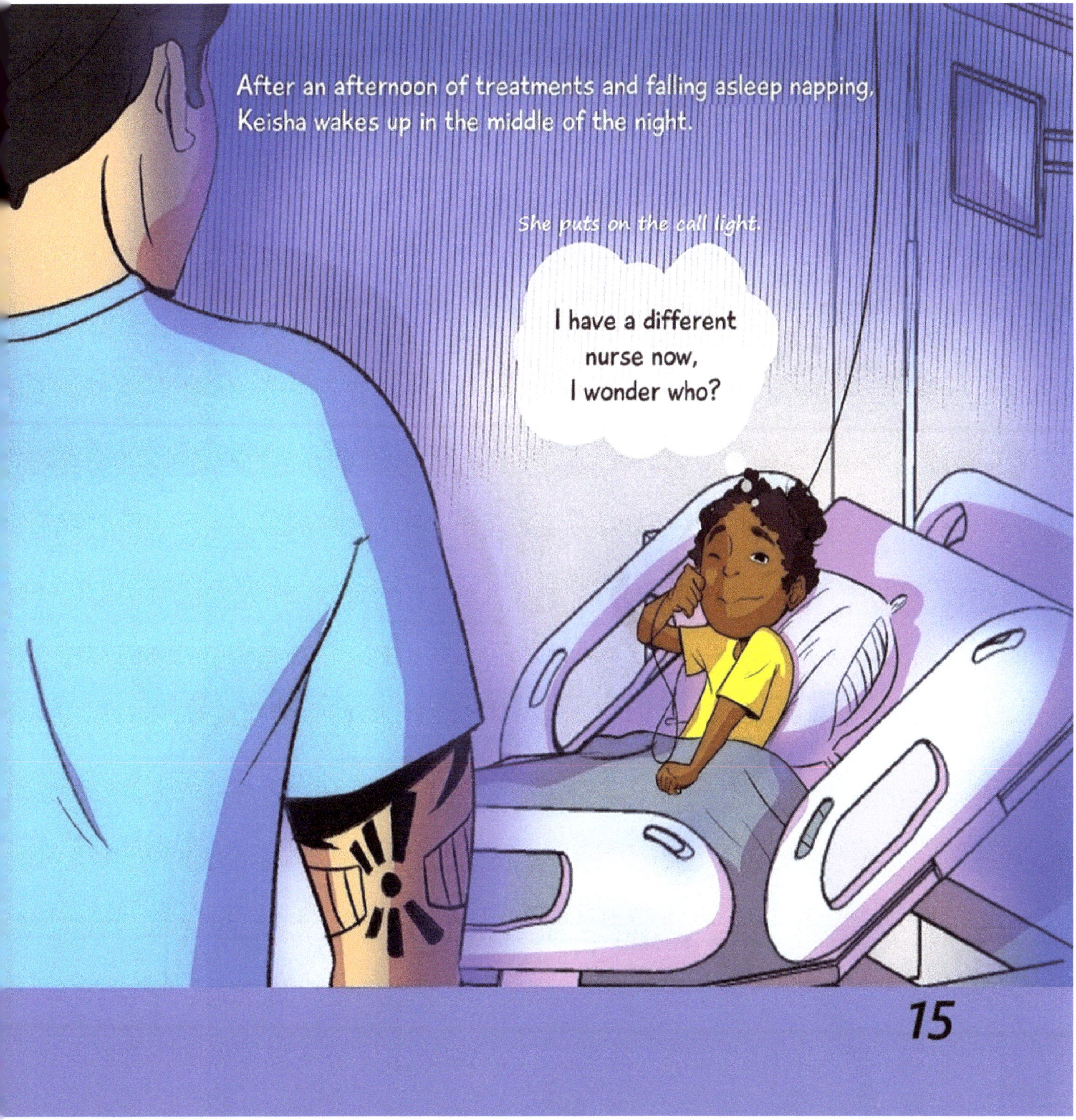

Nurse Ryan answers Keisha's call light and Keisha immediately lights up when she sees it's Ryan.

Ryan! My other favorite nurse!

Hey Keisha! How are you feeling kiddo?

16

Keisha loves to hear Ryan talk about his many tattoos and the stories leading to those tattoos.

Hi Ryan! I feel better now. Do you have any new tattoos to show me?

In fact, I do. This one is in memory of my favorite uncle.

17

Tired from a night of medications, visits from the nurses and respiratory therapists, Keisha falls asleep for a few hours.

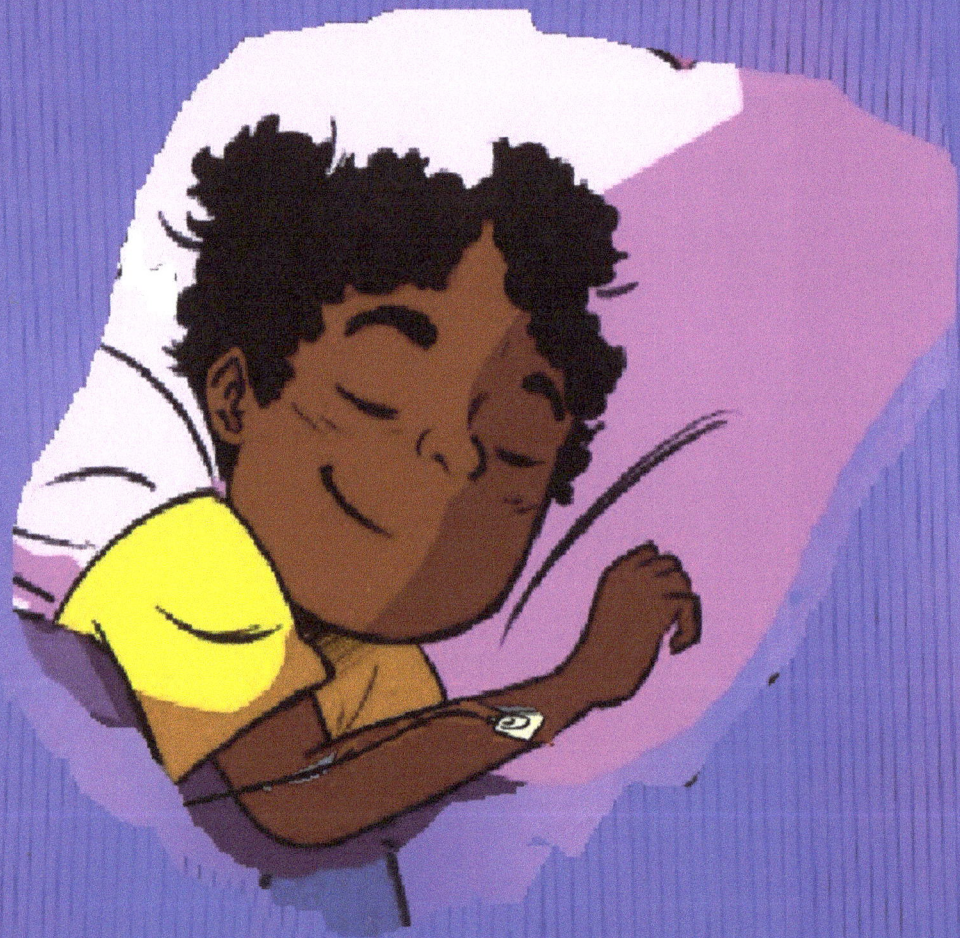

18

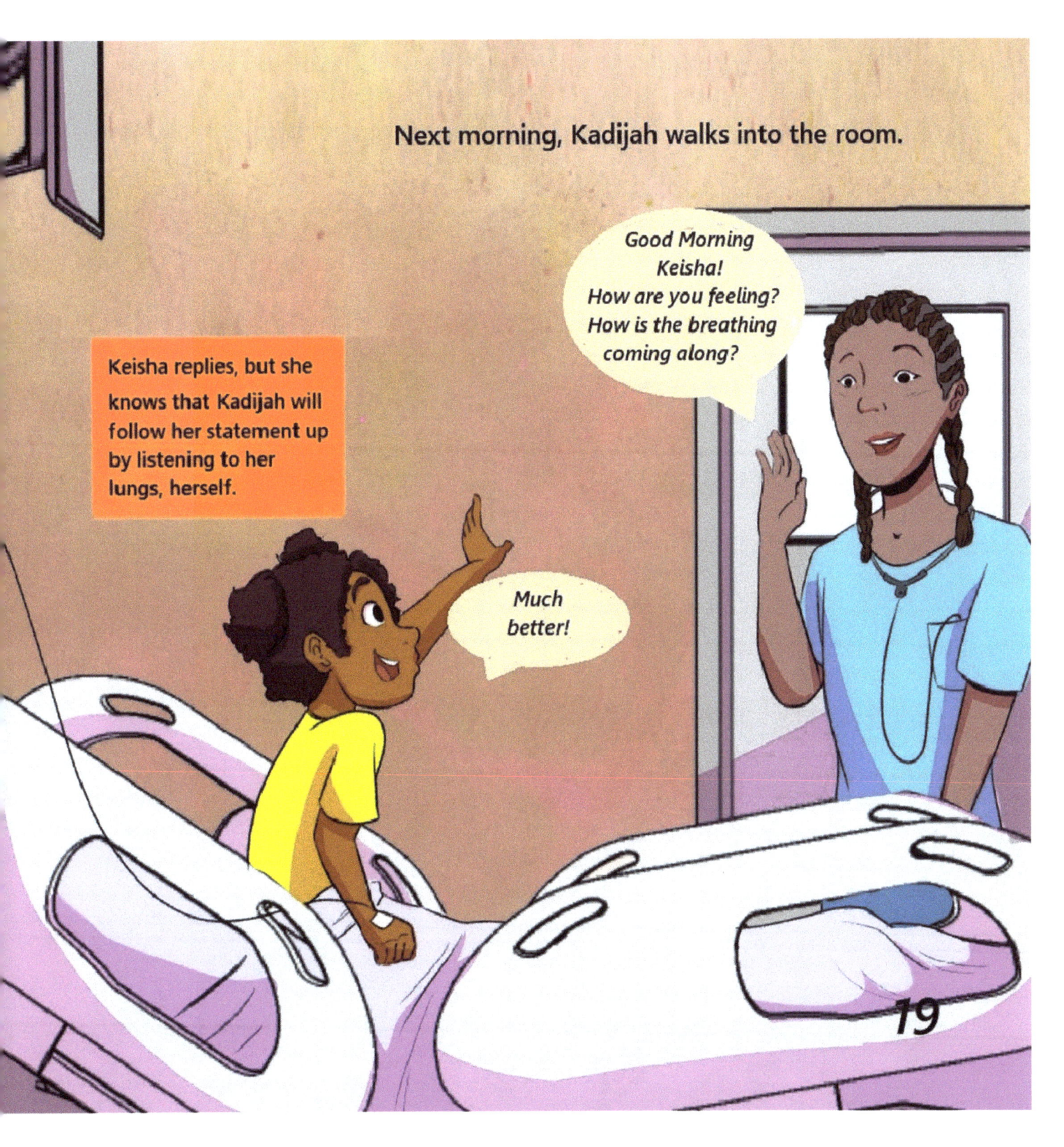

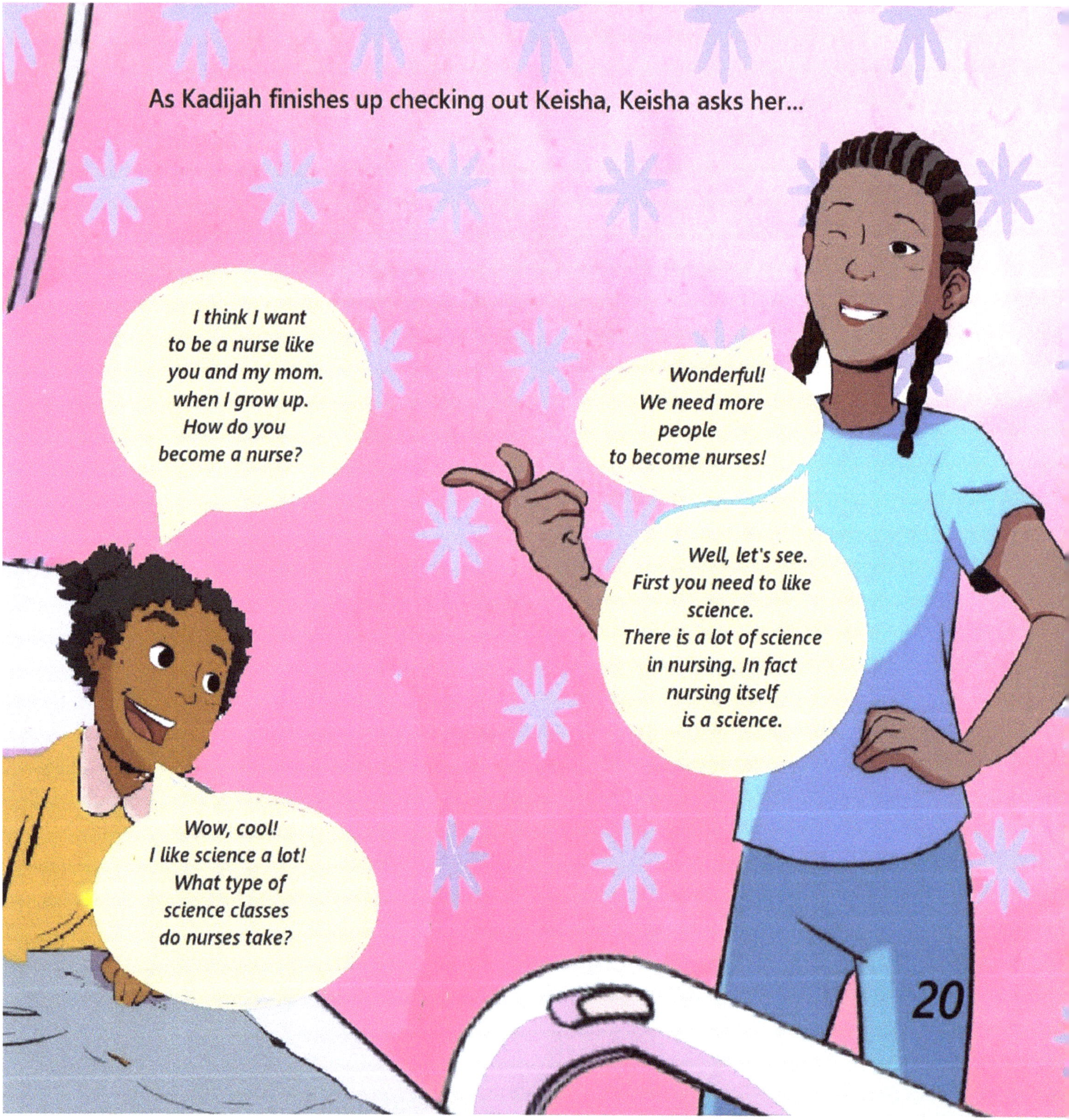
As Kadijah finishes up checking out Keisha, Keisha asks her...
I think I want to be a nurse like you and my mom. when I grow up. How do you become a nurse?
Wonderful! We need more people to become nurses!
Well, let's see. First you need to like science. There is a lot of science in nursing. In fact nursing itself is a science.
Wow, cool! I like science a lot! What type of science classes do nurses take?

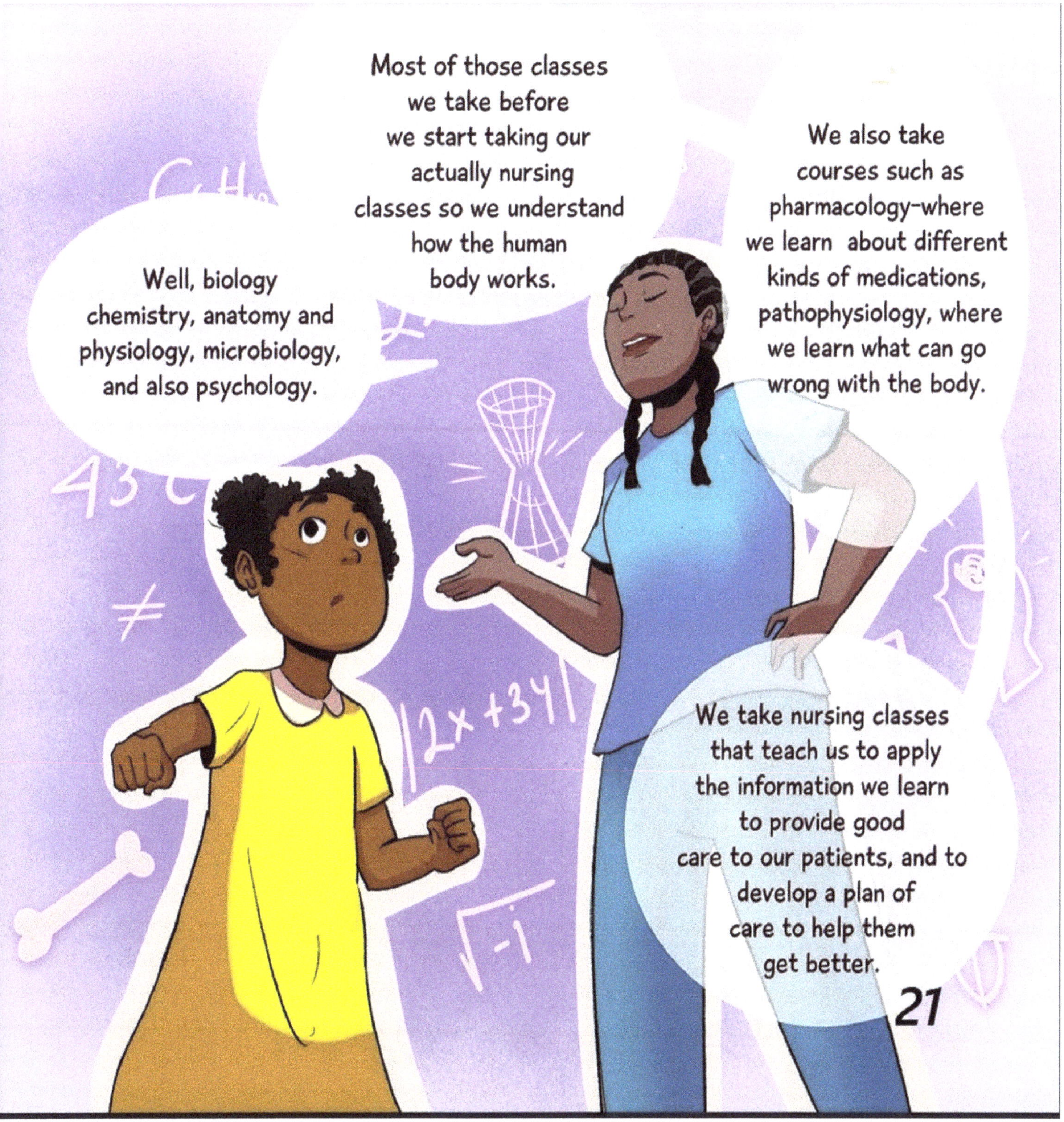
Well, biology chemistry, anatomy and physiology, microbiology, and also psychology.
Most of those classes we take before we start taking our actually nursing classes so we understand how the human body works.
We also take courses such as pharmacology-where we learn about different kinds of medications, pathophysiology, where we learn what can go wrong with the body.
We take nursing classes that teach us to apply the information we learn to provide good care to our patients, and to develop a plan of care to help them get better.

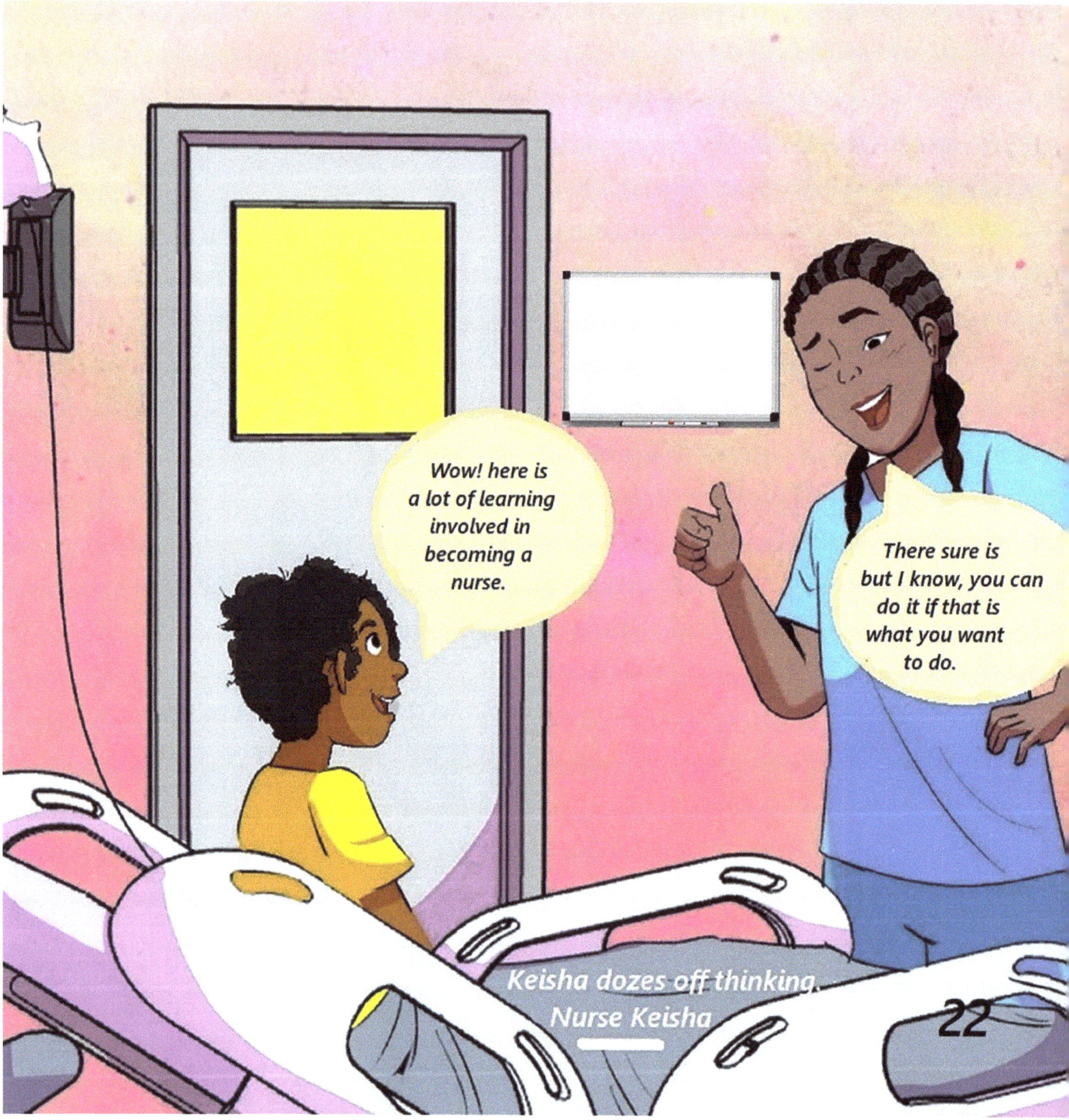
Wow! here is a lot of learning involved in becoming a nurse.
There sure is but I know, you can do it if that is what you want to do.
Keisha dozes off thinking,
Nurse Keisha

When Keisha wakes up, it is around 8 pm. Kadijah's shift has ended. As she wonders who her nurse will be, a nurse walks into the room, and introduces themself as nurse Jo. The nurse's name tag reads, Jo Davis, RN. Keisha is not familiar with this nurse. As the nurse washes their hands and starts to talk to her, Keisha loosens up, and thinks...

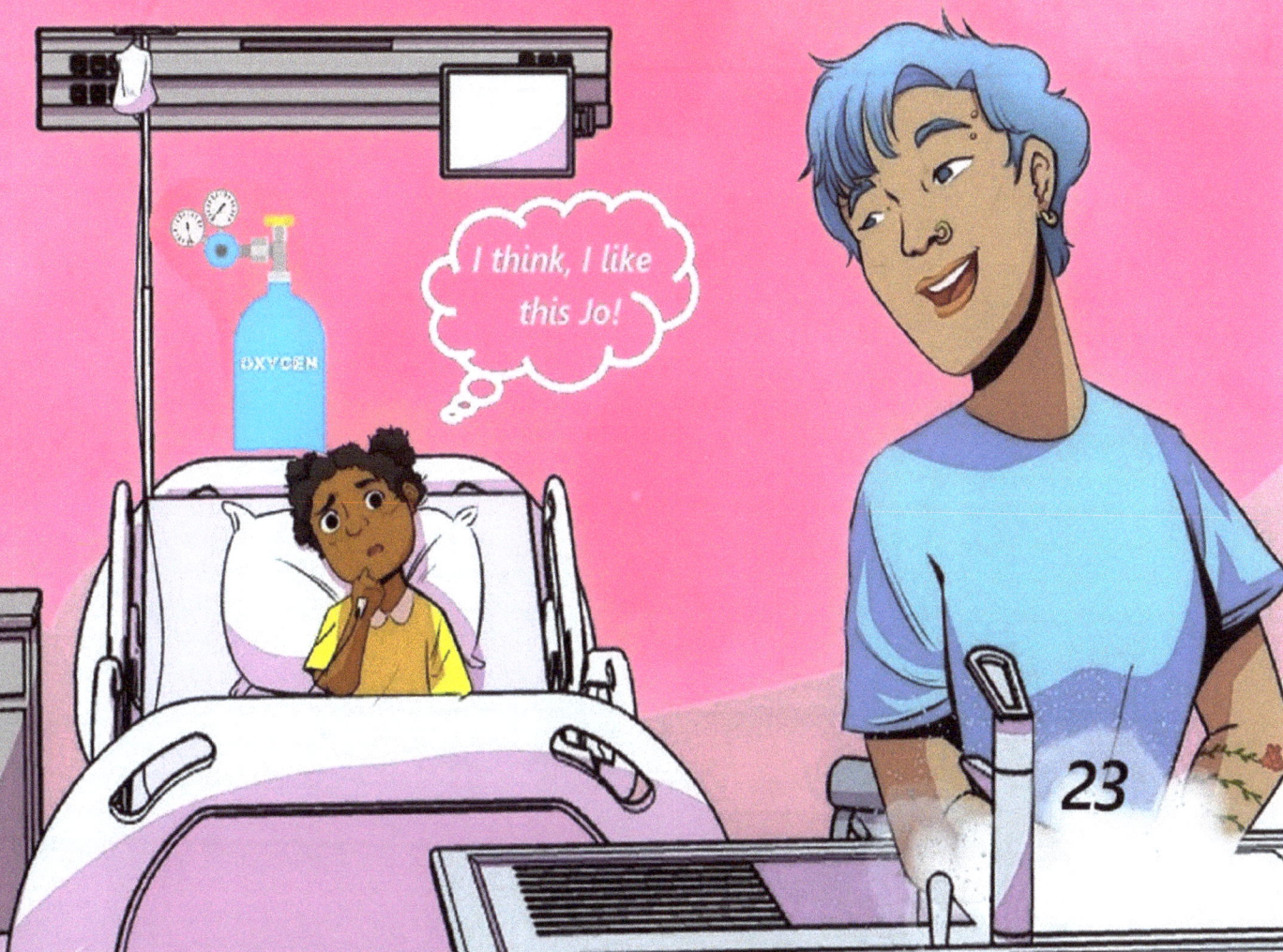

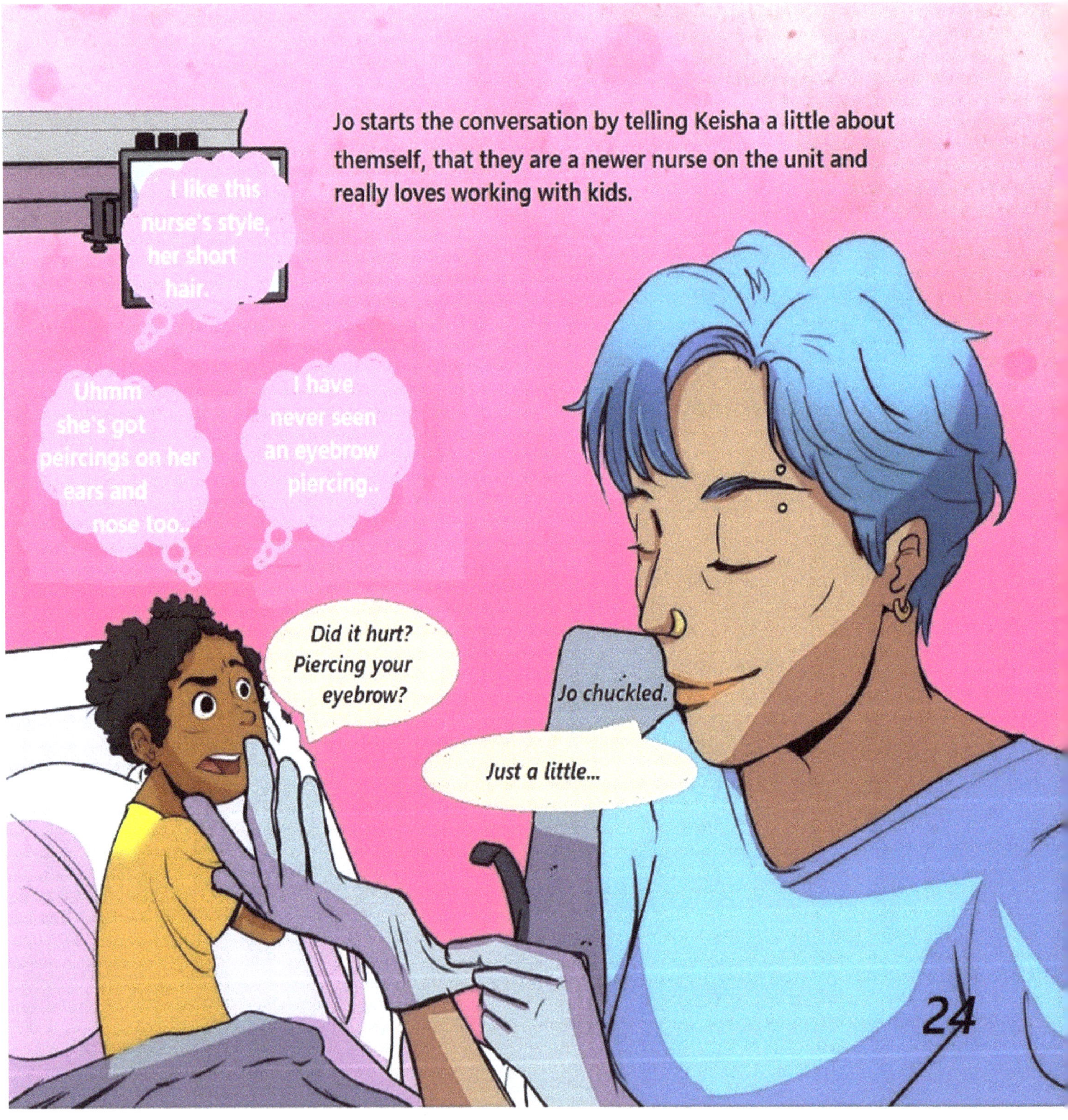
Jo starts the conversation by telling Keisha a little about themself, that they are a newer nurse on the unit and really loves working with kids.
I like this nurse's style, her short hair.
Uhmm she's got peircings on her ears and nose too..
I have never seen an eyebrow piercing..
Did it hurt? Piercing your eyebrow?
Jo chuckled.
Just a little...

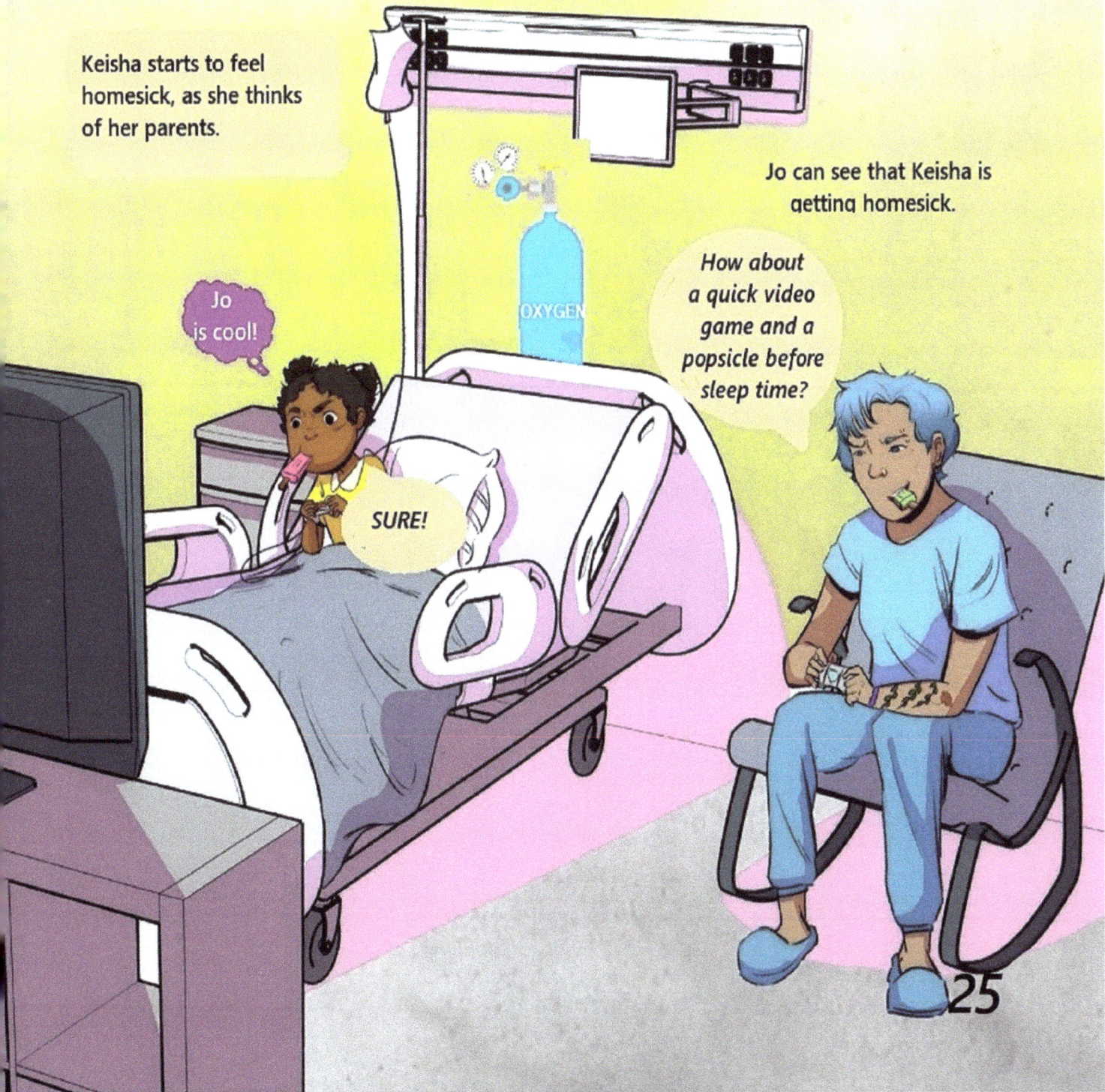

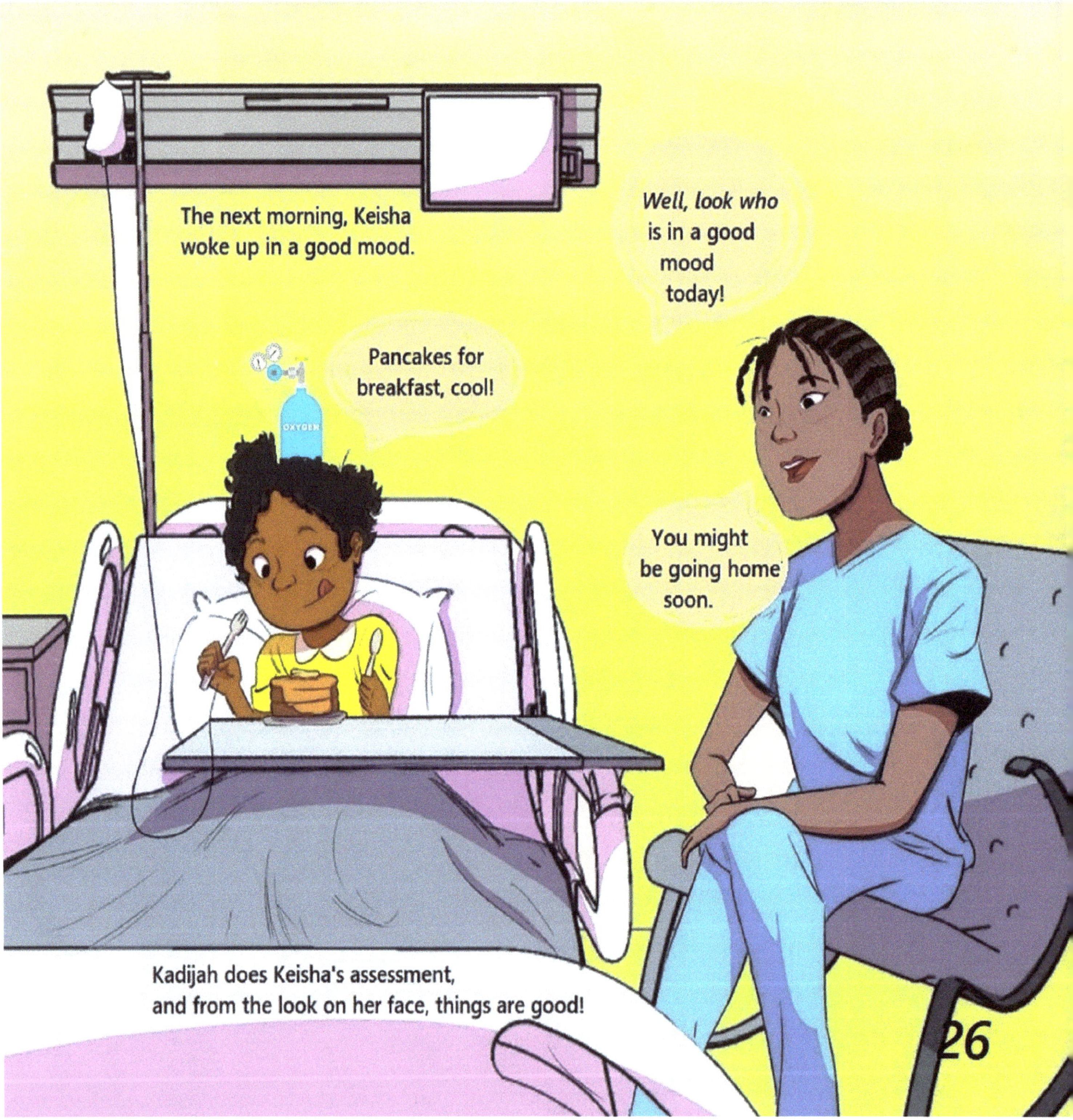
The next morning, Keisha woke up in a good mood.
Pancakes for breakfast, cool!
Well, look who is in a good mood today!
You might be going home soon.
OXYGEN
Kadijah does Keisha's assessment, and from the look on her face, things are good!

Keisha waits until Kadijah has completed her assessment. She wants to talk to Kadijah. She has more questions for Kadijah about nursing school.

I want to be there for people just like you, and Ryan and Jo are there for me. You have been there to make sure I am getting better.

That's what I want to hear!

How long does it take to be a nurse?

It depends on what you want to do. To be a registered nurse like me and your mom, it can take as little as 2 years and as many as 4.

Wow, there is a big difference between 2 and 4 years!

27

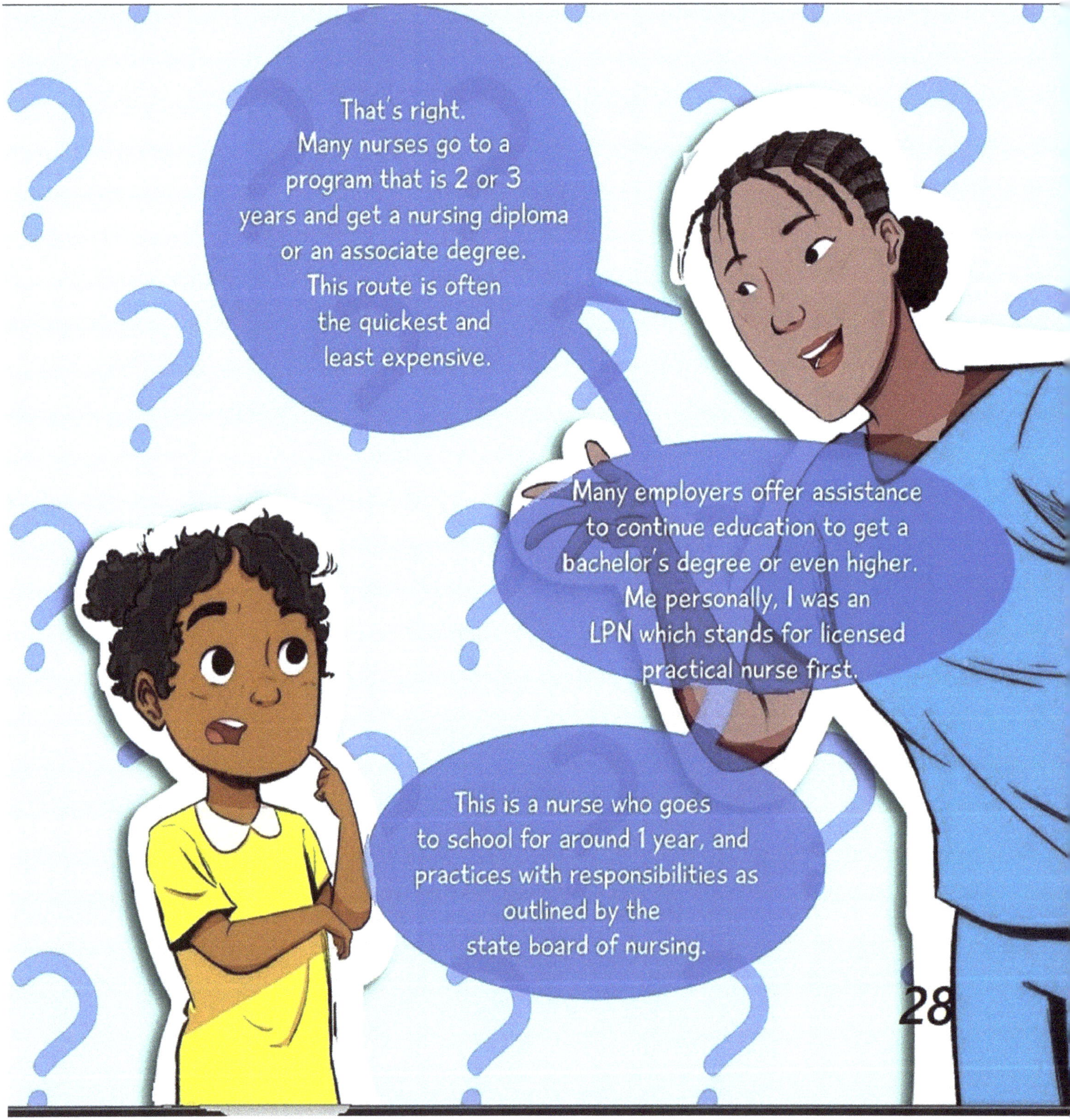
That's right. Many nurses go to a program that is 2 or 3 years and get a nursing diploma or an associate degree. This route is often the quickest and least expensive.
Many employers offer assistance to continue education to get a bachelor's degree or even higher. Me personally, I was an LPN which stands for licensed practical nurse first.
This is a nurse who goes to school for around 1 year, and practices with responsibilities as outlined by the state board of nursing.

I continued on at the same
school in a bridge program to become
a registered nurse, a nurse
with more responsibility, and
then I continued to
get my BSN, and got help
from work to help me
pay for it.

Some people choose to go to
a university from the start and get the
BSN from the beginning, but all RN
program graduate take the same exam
and earn the same starting salary.
I know that is kind of confusing."

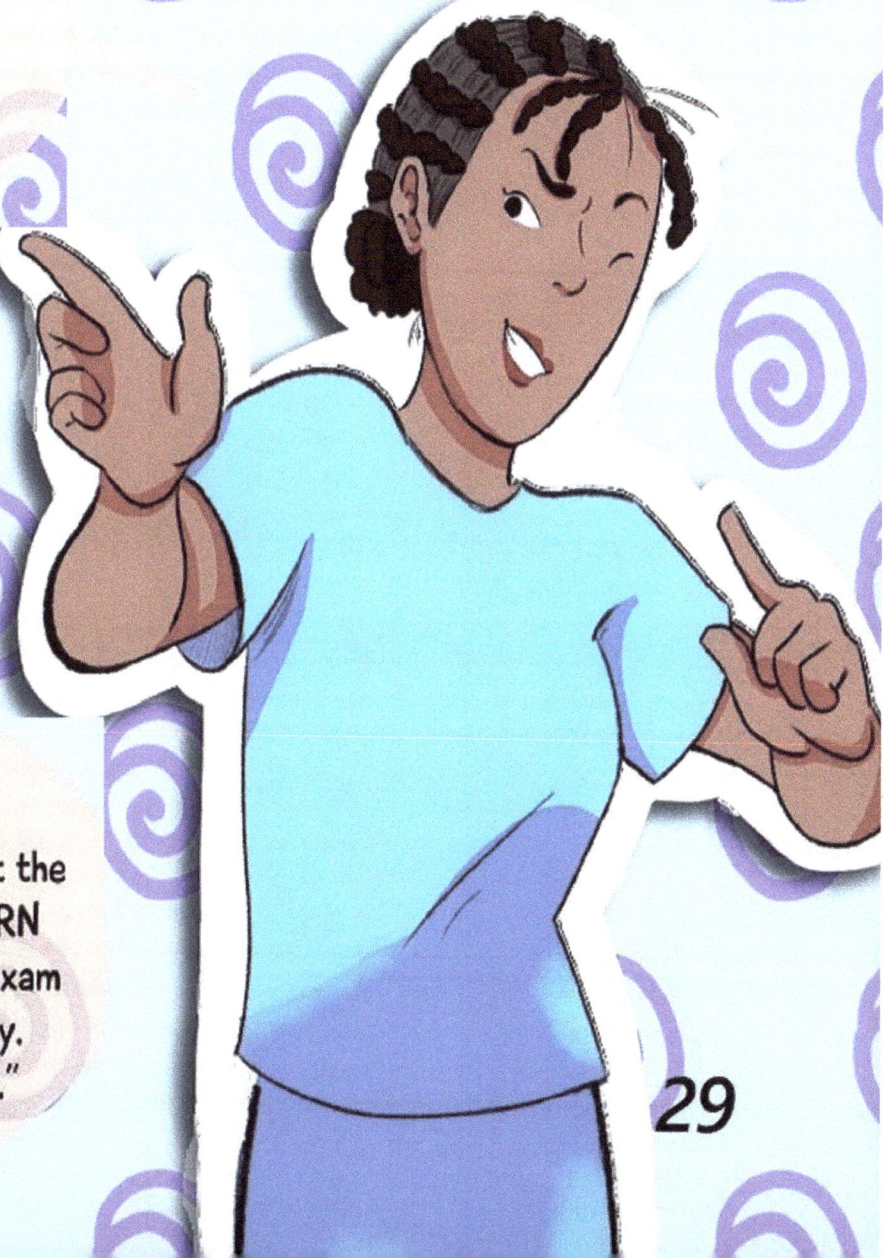

29

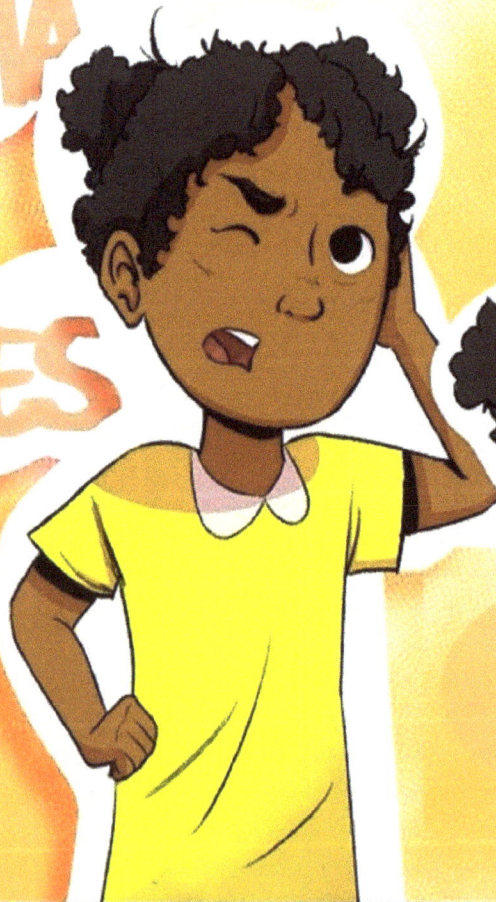

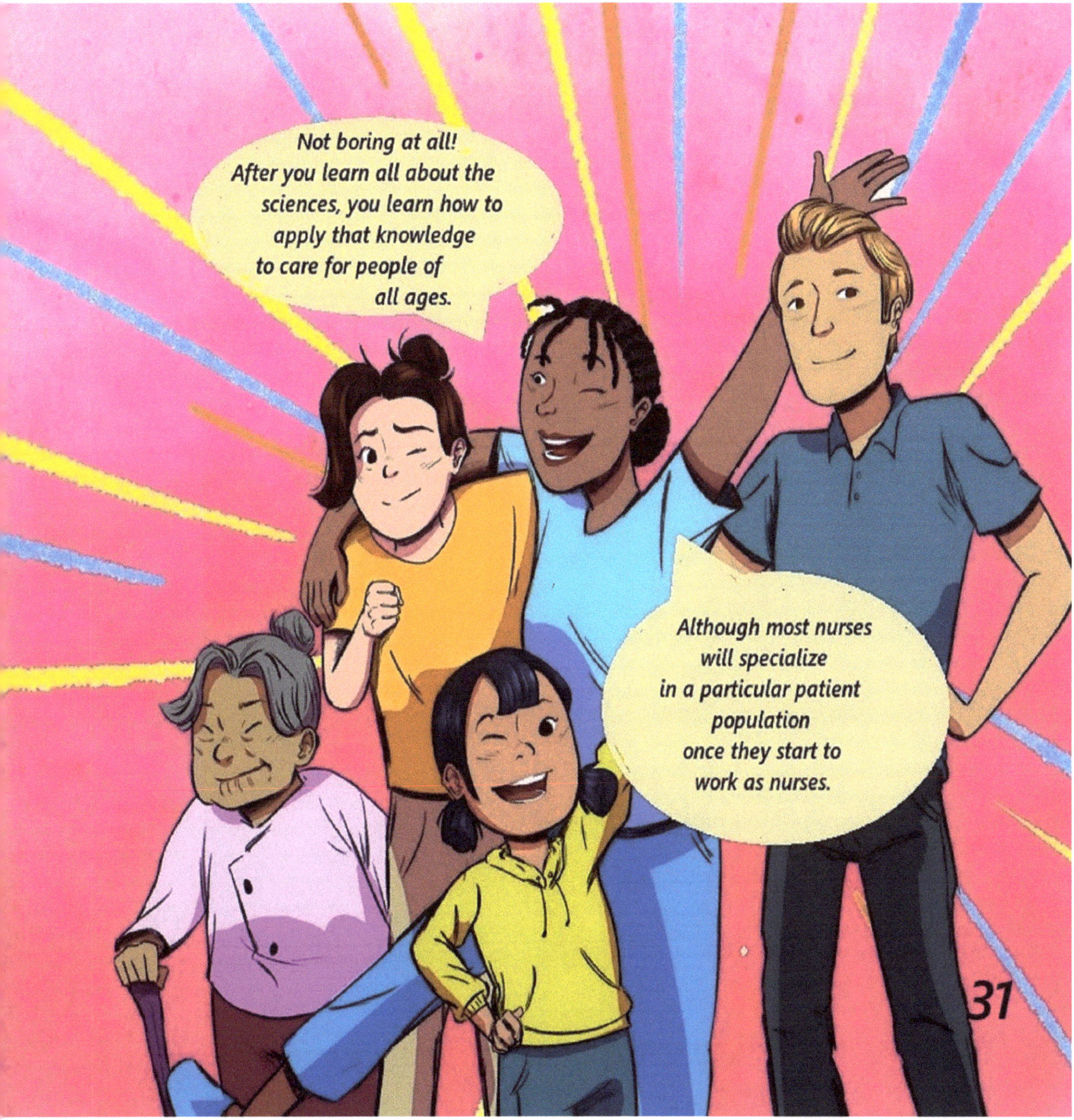
Not boring at all! After you learn all about the sciences, you learn how to apply that knowledge to care for people of all ages.
Although most nurses will specialize in a particular patient population once they start to work as nurses.

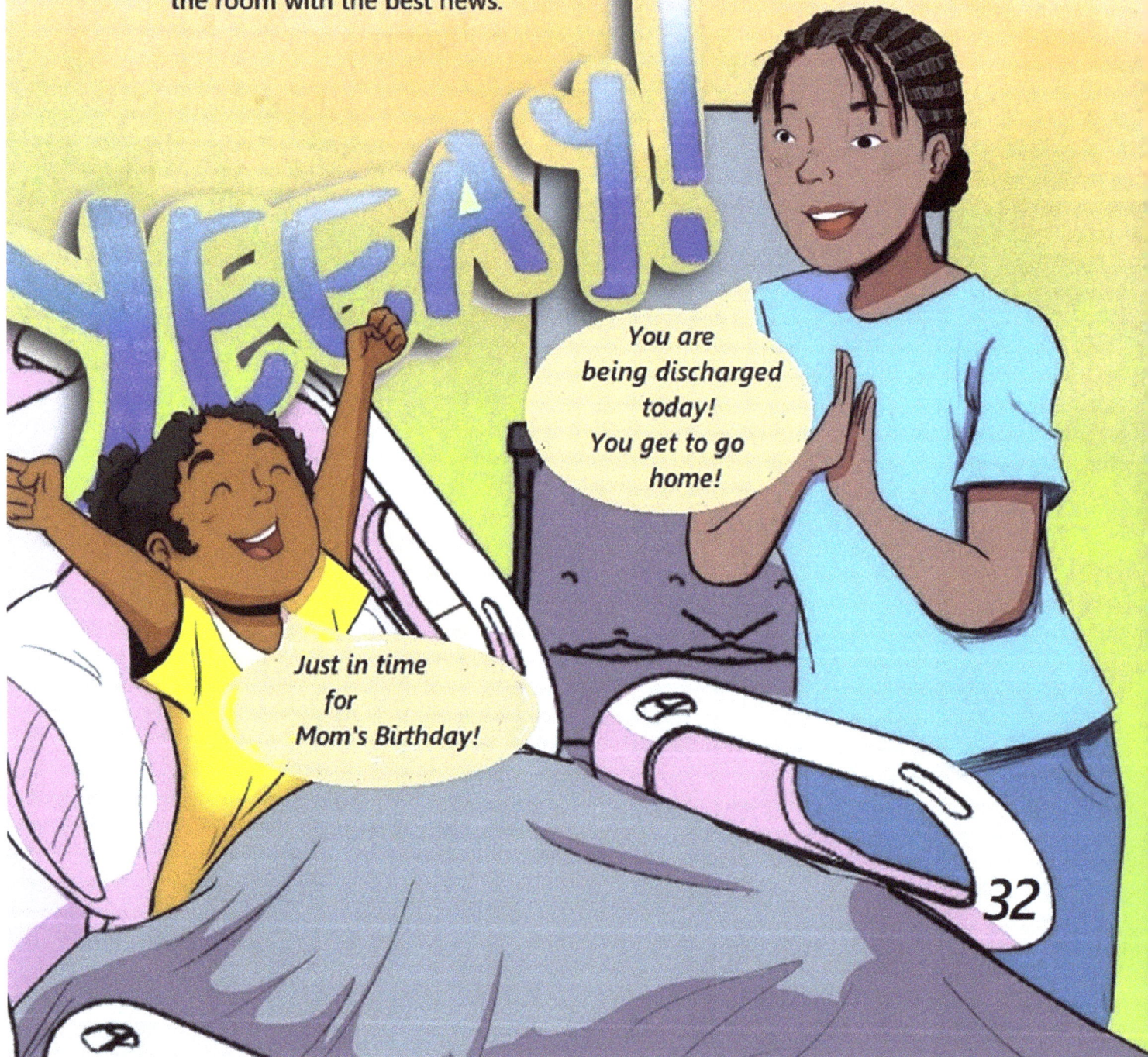

Keisha is so happy to be home, to sleep in her own bed and most of all, to celebrate her mother's birthday!

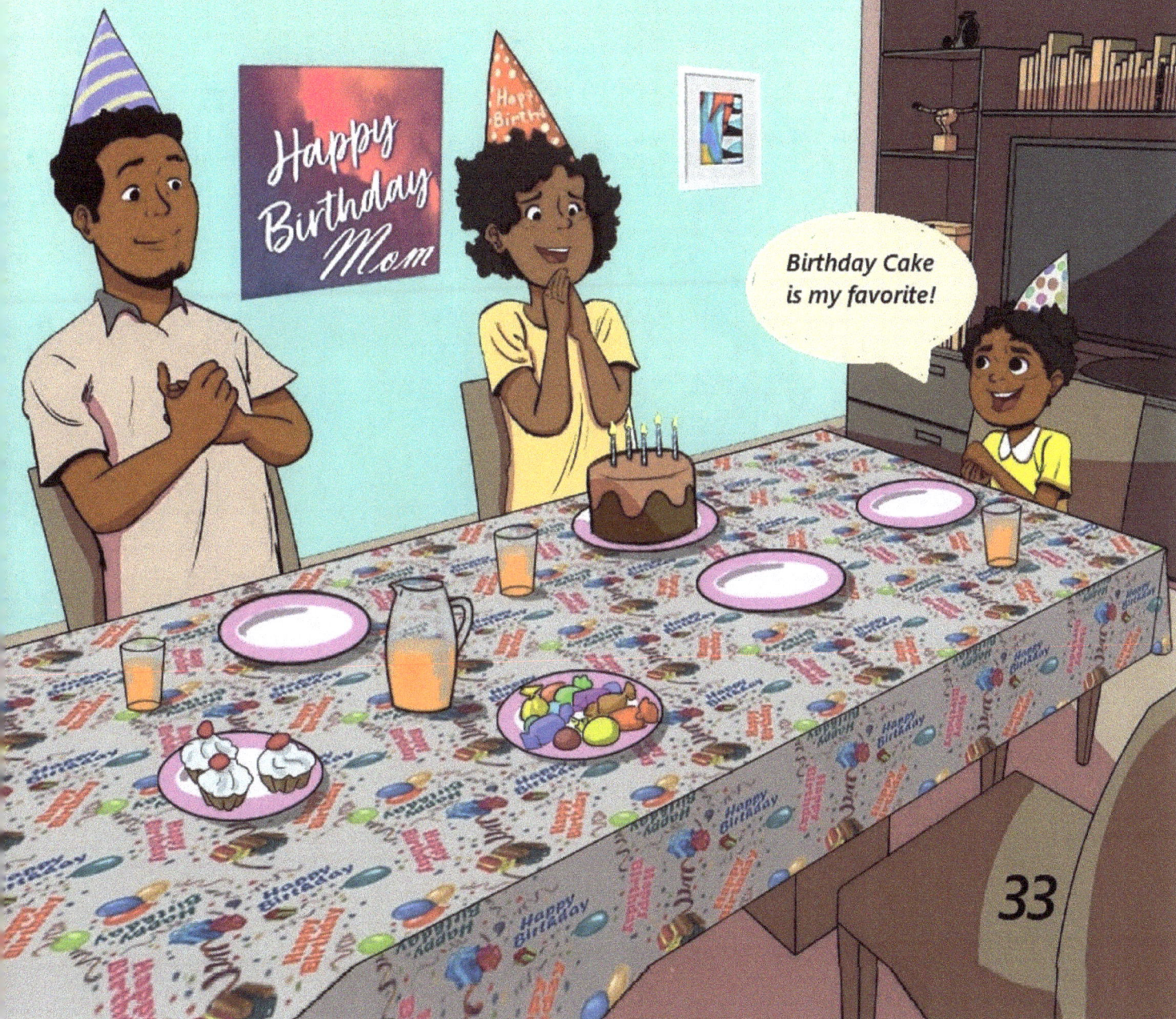

Birthday Cake is my favorite!

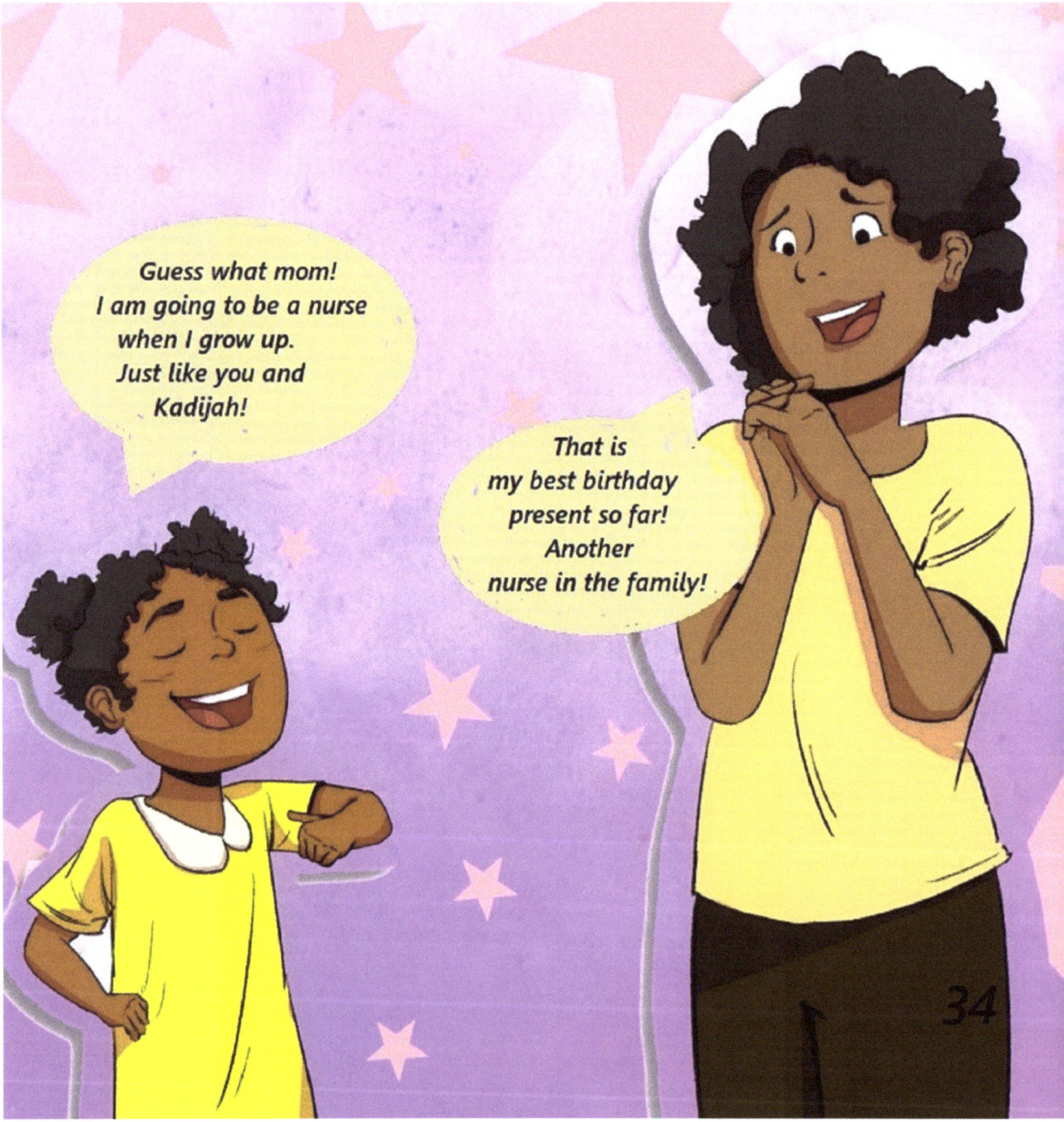
Guess what mom! I am going to be a nurse when I grow up. Just like you and Kadijah!
That is my best birthday present so far! Another nurse in the family!

Later on that night, as Keisha falls asleep after an exhausting day, Keisha dreams of herself all grown up as a nurse working with kids with asthma just like her.

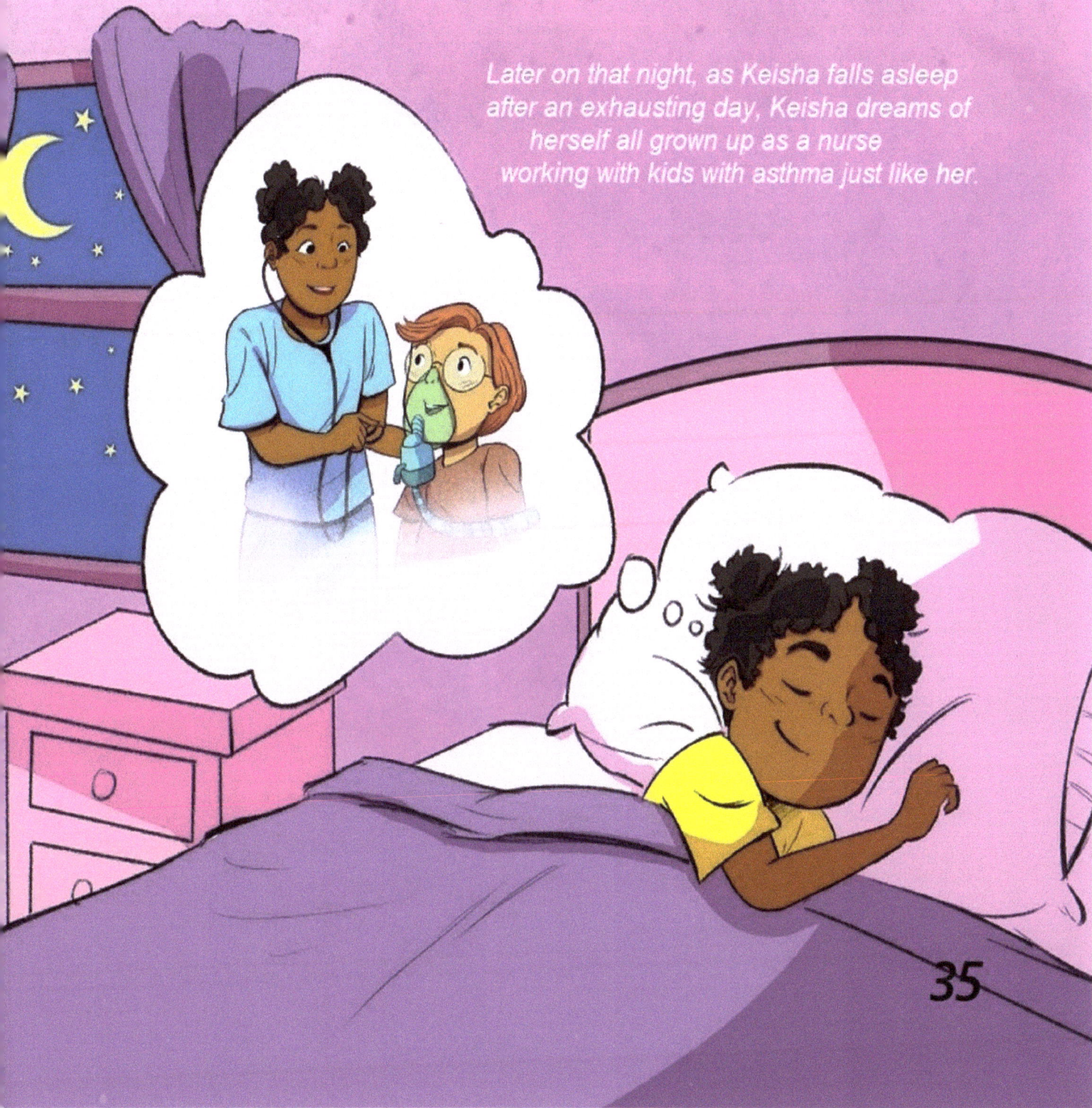

35

Why Keisha Wanted to Become a NURSE

About the Author

Glossary Of Important Words Used In The Story

Asthma – is an illness affecting the airways in the lungs. These airways are tubes that bring air in and out of the lungs. When a person has asthma, the airways can become irritated and they can become narrow, making it hard for air to get out when a person breathes. NIH, 2022

Assessment-the process of gathering information

Emergency department -part of a hospital that offers 24 hour medical care

Inhaler - a handheld device used to deliver medication that assists with breathing to the lungs.

IV – a tube inserted into a vein to give medications or fluids

Lungs – spongy, pinkish gray organ that take in oxygen through the process of breathing

Medications – a herb or chemical compound used to treat an illness or condition

Respiratory therapist —works under the direction of a doctor to help patients who are having trouble breathing

Stethoscope is a tool used by people who work in health care to hear how certain parts of the body are functioning. It is comprised of a disc-shaped piece that is placed on the person's skin, tubing that conducts the sound, and ear pieces to listen. The tool can be used to listen to various parts of the body including but not limited to the lungs, abdomen (belly), heart, etc.

Other Useful Words To Know

Call light • Science • Chemistry • Anatomy • Microbiology

Physiology • Psychology • Pharmacology • Pathophysiology

Plan of care • Shift • Patient population • Discharged

Dr. Clary-Muronda

has been a nurse for over 30 years. A Philadelphia native from the West Oak Lane section of the city, she attended Albert Einstein School of Nursing, and continued on with her education over the years and later earned a PhD in Nursing Science from the Medical University of South Carolina in Charleston. She enjoys teaching undergraduate nursing students, mentoring young students who aspire to work in the health professions, and inspiring nurses to be the best they can be.

www.ingramcontent.com/pod-product-compliance
Lightning Source LLC
Chambersburg PA
CBHW042348030426
42335CB00031B/3494

* 9 7 8 1 9 6 5 3 9 8 3 7 1 *